D1123352

Surviving After Cancer

Surviving After Cancer

Living the New Normal

Anne Katz

ROWMAN & LITTLEFIELD PUBLISHERS, INC.
Lanham • Boulder • New York • Toronto • Plymouth, UK

Published by Rowman & Littlefield Publishers, Inc.
A wholly owned subsidiary of The Rowman & Littlefield Publishing Group, Inc.
4501 Forbes Boulevard, Suite 200, Lanham, Maryland 20706
http://www.rowmanlittlefield.com

Estover Road, Plymouth PL6 7PY, United Kingdom

British Library Cataloguing in Publication Information Available

Library of Congress Cataloging-in-Publication Data

Katz, Anne.
  Surviving after cancer : living the new normal / Anne Katz.
    p. cm.
  Includes bibliographical references and index.
  ISBN 978-1-4422-0365-5 (cloth : alk. paper) — ISBN 978-1-4422-0367-9 (electronic)
  1. Cancer—Popular works. 2. Cancer—Patients—Popular works. I. Title.
  RC263.K277 2011
  616.99'4—dc22   2010043444

Printed in the United States of America

Always, Alan

Contents

Part I: What Is the New Normal?

1 You're a Survivor Now   3

Part II: The Challenges of Being a Cancer Survivor

2 Is the Cancer Back?   9
3 When Will I Be Happy Again?   27
4 What Will Everyone Say?   45
5 Why Do I Feel So Tired?   63
6 Where Did That Feeling Go?   83
7 Feeling Fit   103
8 What Should I Be Looking For?   119
9 We Want to Start a Family   131
10 Am I Losing My Mind?   151

Part III: Surviving and Thriving: The New Normal

11 A Blueprint for Health   171
12 Resources   189

Bibliography   201
Index   207
About the Author   209

Part I

WHAT IS THE NEW NORMAL?

• 1 •

You're a Survivor Now

$\mathcal{C}$ancer survivor." What does that mean? How do you know if you are one? Is there some magical sign that heralds your arrival at a place you've never been before? How does it feel? Are your worries over? Will side effects of treatment magically disappear and life go back to what it was before? This chapter sets the stage for the rest of the book by explaining this new phase of the cancer journey and by identifying common challenges for the years of healthy living that hopefully lie ahead.

Cancer survivorship is a relatively new term for a distinct phase of the cancer experience. A report from the President's Cancer Panel in 2004 attempted to define this term:

> Among health professionals, people with a cancer history, and the public, views differ as to when a person with cancer becomes a survivor. Many consider a person to be a survivor from the moment of diagnosis; in recent years, this view has become increasingly prevalent. Some, however, think that a person with a cancer diagnosis cannot be considered a survivor until he or she completes initial treatment. Others believe a person with cancer can be considered a survivor if he or she lives 5 years beyond diagnosis. Still others believe survivorship begins at some other point after diagnosis and treatment, and some reject the term "survivor" entirely, preferring to think of people with a cancer history as fighters, "thrivers," champions, patients, or simply as individuals who have had a life-threatening disease. A considerable number of people with a cancer history maintain that they will have survived cancer if they die from another cause.

There are other ways of looking at survivorship. The Office of Cancer Survivorship at the National Cancer Institutes states their definition in the following manner: "An individual is considered a cancer survivor from the time of diagnosis, through the balance of his or her life. Family members, friends, and caregivers are also impacted by the survivorship experience and are therefore included in this definition." However, the Office of Cancer Survivorship decided to focus its research on the period after diagnosis and treatment.

Fitzhugh Mullan, a cancer survivor and founding member of the National Coalition for Cancer Survivorship, describes three seasons of survival: the first is acute survival that begins with diagnosis and continues through active treatment. The second is that of extended survival, which begins with the termination of active treatment and a period of disease remission. The third is permanent survival or cure.

But what about those who have completed active treatment and are prescribed adjuvant treatment? Women with breast cancer fall into this category. Many will take antiestrogen medication for years following surgery, radiation, and chemotherapy. Are they survivors or still in active treatment? And what about men who are diagnosed with prostate cancer and opt for deferred treatment by following an active surveillance protocol? They don't have surgery or radiation, so are they ever regarded as survivors?

Confused? Well, so are many health care providers! Despite the confusion over terminology and definitions, there is a lot of ongoing research and service provision for people who have had cancer. Chapter 12 contains a list of organizations and their websites that provide useful information for cancer survivors and their families. There is also a list of books that you may find helpful and informative.

And what about this book? In the following nine chapters, you will read about nine individuals who have had different kinds of cancer and are facing various challenges. From my clinical experience and a detailed review of the literature, there are several issues that affect cancer survivors. The following chapters address these important issues.

In chapter 2, you will read about Nancy, a forty-five-year-old woman who was treated for breast cancer. Nancy is struggling with the fear that the cancer will come back. This fear of recurrence is common and can be debilitating—some cancer survivors live every day with high anxiety that interferes with their ability to function. Nancy finds it difficult to ask for help in dealing with her anxiety, but she eventually finds some relief through the practice of mindfulness meditation.

Another common challenge after treatment is feeling depressed. In chapter 3, you will meet Robert, a colon cancer survivor. When his chemotherapy is over, he begins to feel depressed and hopeless. He tries to hide it from his wife, but eventually one of the nurses notices how down he is and offers him help in the form of a referral to a psychiatrist. Despite some initial resistance, Robert finds that antidepressants begin to improve his mood.

Going back to work can be a significant challenge after months of treatment. In chapter 4, you will learn how Steve, a construction worker, is able to go back to work despite some lingering side effects from prostate cancer surgery. This chapter highlights some of the legislation in place to help cancer survivors reenter the work force, as well as some of the challenges facing people in the workplace.

Fatigue is another challenge for cancer survivors. Many people assume that once treatment is over they will instantly go back to feeling normal again. Barb's story in chapter 5 illustrates some of the persistent issues for cancer survivors. Six months after completing treatment for uterine cancer, she still feels exhausted and is frustrated by her lack of energy. She is surprised when she learns that getting regular exercise will help combat the fatigue.

An often unspoken side effect of all cancer treatments is the effect on sexuality and sexual functioning. In chapter 6, you will meet Karen and Gary, who experience some fairly typical challenges after Karen goes into menopause after a stem cell transplant. The couple doesn't talk about what is happening, and they start to live separate lives. Eventually Karen goes to an information session about menopause, where she hears a sex therapist talk about some of the difficulties that couples face when hormonal changes affect their sex life.

In chapter 7, you will learn about the benefits of a healthy diet and exercise through the story of Morrie, an older man with bladder cancer. His wife Esther is determined to help him lead a healthier life, and she enlists the help of their children and grandchildren in her quest. Making lifestyle changes is always difficult, and Morrie's story highlights the evidence for the benefits of diet and exercise in survivorship.

An important task of the survivorship phase is keeping up with medical appointments and having needed tests done on schedule. It is also important to know the details of the kind of cancer you had and the treatments that were performed. One way of making sure you have all of this information is to have a document called a Survivorship Care Plan. The details about this are explained in the story of Sue, a young woman who had cancer as a teenager and who is now interested in finding out more about her cancer history.

Many cancer survivors have not started or completed childbearing when the cancer diagnosis is made—this can present some significant challenges. In chapter 9, you will meet David and Lesley, who are one such couple. When Lesley was diagnosed with cancer, their only thought was to save her life. Now that she is well again, they want to have a baby, but they have some obstacles to face.

In the final story of this book, you will learn about Gail's struggle with some cognitive changes related to her medication. Gail is a nurse on a busy medical ward who encounters difficulty with her memory and her ability to concentrate. This affects her work and causes her great distress. With the help of her oncologist and a human resources staff person, Gail is able to make changes that allow her to return to work.

The last two chapters provide specific information and resources for the cancer survivor and his or her family. Chapter 11 provides an overview of strategies and suggestions for living well during the years after treatment. Information that has been presented as part of the survivors' stories is reviewed here so that readers may have a concise and focused understanding of the nine key issues in survivorship. Chapter 12 provides the reader with additional information about strategies that are suggested to help the survivor, as well as resources, websites, and books to further enhance your understanding about how to live well during the survivorship phase.

Cancer changes everything. Anyone who has been through it as a patient or family member will attest to that. But what comes after cancer—the new normal—can be healthier and happier than what used to be. The new normal is a revamp of the old normal, a chance to engage in life with a heart full of hope and a mind full of information.

Part II

THE CHALLENGES OF BEING A CANCER SURVIVOR

· 2 ·

Is the Cancer Back?

The number-one fear of most cancer survivors is that the cancer will come back. In this chapter, you will meet Nancy, a forty-five-year-old woman who was treated for breast cancer. Nancy struggles every day to overcome her fear that the cancer is coming back.

Nancy was diagnosed with breast cancer almost three years ago. She had just had her third and last baby, a little girl named Emma, who was a surprise. Nancy was forty years old, and when she missed a couple of periods, she thought she was entering menopause. But the fatigue and nausea that overwhelmed her were suspicious, and almost as a joke she bought a home pregnancy test. It was positive! Nancy was both happy and also a little embarrassed; her two other children, Grace and Juliet, were teenagers already. How could this happen to her? Her husband Tim was as proud as a peacock. He had always wanted more children, four or five, and even this late in their lives, another baby would be a blessing.

Nancy's pregnancy went smoothly. She had a little bit of a problem with her blood pressure right at the end, but on a sunny June day, baby Emma joined their family. Grace and Juliet waited outside the delivery room and held Emma within moments of her birth. Any embarrassment they might have felt while their mom was pregnant disappeared the moment they held the tiny baby in their arms. She was so pretty, her big gray eyes staring at their faces as if she already knew them, and her tiny hands like starfish reaching out to touch their faces. It was love at first sight for the whole family. Emma was a good baby; she hardly cried, and when she did, there were four eager people to hold her.

Nancy was breast-feeding, and this was an unexpected gift of being an older new mother. With both of the older girls, she had to go back to work

9

within four weeks of their births and so bottle-fed them from the beginning. She was not working when she had Emma, so she had all the time in the world to breast-feed, rest, and enjoy the new baby. One day, as she removed Emma from her breast after a very long feed, she noticed a small lump on the side of her breast. For an instant, a flicker of fear passed over her heart, but she shook her head. It was probably just a lump from a milk gland, she reassured herself. But over the next week, it was still there, an increasing worry in her otherwise happy life.

She had to take Emma for her six-week visit to the doctor, and while they were there, Nancy mentioned to Dr. Glass that she had felt this lump on her right breast. Dr. Glass did not seem concerned but suggested that she take a look at it. Her face was creased in concentration as she gently and then more firmly felt Nancy's breast.

"I don't want to worry you, Nancy," she said, "but I'm just not sure that it's nothing. I want you to have a mammogram just to be sure."

Nancy's heart skipped a beat, and a sick feeling swept over her. She didn't even have to wait for the results of the many tests she had over the next week. She just knew. It was breast cancer, and within three weeks she had surgery to remove her breast. She had been offered less invasive surgery to remove just the lump, but she wanted to be sure the cancer was gone. Six weeks after the surgery, she started chemotherapy. The whole experience was just a blur. Tim had taken an extended leave from work to be with Emma, and the older girls were a tremendous help. She couldn't even hold Emma for the first four weeks after the surgery, and during the weeks of chemotherapy, she was just too sick and exhausted to do anything for the baby. Emma seemed oblivious to the changes in her young life. She grew and developed according to some internal clock. She was a happy baby, willing to accept a bottle from anyone, but she preferred her dad to change her diapers. Her sisters liked that task least of all, and she probably knew that. They were happy to bathe her and carry her around, and she was a big hit with their friends.

Breast cancer is rare in women during the childbearing years. Pregnancy conveys a slight increase in the risk of developing breast cancer, but usually for just a few years. This may be due to changes in hormone levels during pregnancy. The risk of being diagnosed with breast cancer increases with age, and Nancy was forty when she was pregnant with her third baby. Her decision to have a mastectomy was a personal one. Many women opt for a lumpectomy (removal of the lump only), which is usually followed by radiation to the affected breast. Because she had not yet gone through menopause when her breast cancer was detected, Nancy also had chemotherapy, which has been shown to reduce the risk of the cancer recurring.

Life eventually went back to some sort of normal after Nancy's chemotherapy was over. She was weak and tired and had no hair. She also had little interest in what was going on around her. Tim was worried that she was depressed, but she was emphatic in telling him that she just needed to rest. He listened, and she did get better. But it took almost another six months before she was her old self. She didn't talk much about her feelings at the best of times, and she seemed to fill her days with taking care of Emma. She told Tim that she didn't want to go back to work ever, that she needed to make up time with little Emma, and Tim agreed.

During that time, Emma had grown into a toddler, an energetic and curious little girl who was starting to talk like a teenager under her sisters' influence. Grace and Juliet were young women now. Grace was in her sophomore year of college and planned to find work in a nearby city so she could be close to home. Juliet was now eighteen years old and had grown into a quietly confident young woman who excelled in all kinds of sport. She was starting college in the fall and had decided to go to the state college in their hometown so that she too could be close to her parents and Emma.

It can take a long time to recover from the effects of both surgery and chemotherapy. Many cancer patients and their families think that the day the treatment is over, they will be their normal selves again. This can lead to frustration on the part of both the patient and their family. It is normal to be weak and tired after the long weeks of chemotherapy. If your hair has fallen out, it will gradually start to grow back, but this may serve as a reminder of the challenges of treatment.

Nancy found herself thinking about what had happened more and more as the months and then years went by. It had all been a bit of a blur—the surprise pregnancy, then finding the lump so soon after the baby was born, and then the surgery followed by months of chemotherapy. She dreaded visiting any of the doctors, and there were so many visits! She had to see the oncologist every three months, and for days before each appointment she couldn't sleep. She dreaded what would happen at the appointment. Even the thought of entering the building made her nervous. She hated the smell of the place and the bright lights and waiting in the crowded waiting room made her heart beat so fast she thought it would fly out of her chest. She hated seeing all the other patients waiting, their bald heads covered by a variety of scarves and hats. Just seeing them made her pat her head for reassurance that her hair had grown back, even though it had grown back just as thick as it had always been. She even dreaded going to have her blood tests a few days before seeing the oncologist. She would watch the red blood flow into the test tube, and she was sure she could see cancer cells swirling in the blood. Part of her knew this was just a fantasy, but in the moment, she was really convinced. It was not until the doctor said the words, "Everything is fine, Nancy. The cancer is not back," that she could relax. Until the next visit, that is.

———⚬⚬⚬———

It is quite common for the period of treatment to be a blur that you cannot quite remember. And it is also quite normal to have some lingering feelings of fear when you have to go back to where you were treated. The cancer center may be a place about which you have mostly bad or painful memories. That is okay. But follow-up care for your cancer is part of being a cancer survivor, and coming to terms with your feelings and trying to make peace with them is an important task.

———⚬⚬⚬———

Nancy continued to think about the cancer. It was strange. The thoughts came more and more often, and she had no control over them. She would be playing with Emma in the yard, and suddenly something would pop into her head. In the beginning, she thought a lot about the cancer coming back and what it would feel like when the doctor told her it was back. She imagined her hands going cold and her heart starting to beat faster. And sitting in the bright sunshine as Emma played in the grass, she would feel her heart beating faster, and her hands would get cold. She could bring herself back to reality after a few minutes, but while she was thinking about it, it was as if it were actually happening. Then she started thinking about having more chemotherapy if the cancer was back. She would start to breathe faster as she thought about the needles and the pills and feeling sick and weak. These images and feelings were even worse than thinking about hearing that the cancer was back.

———⚬⚬⚬———

What Nancy is experiencing is called "intrusive thoughts." They are thoughts, usually of a painful or frightening nature, that pop into your head. They seem to occur quite randomly, with nothing obvious that prompts them. They can cause physical symptoms such as faster heartbeat or rapid breathing, and they can even cause a full-blown panic attack.

———⚬⚬⚬———

At first she didn't tell anyone that she was having these thoughts. She didn't want to worry Tim, who was stressed about work. She couldn't talk to the girls about it, either. So she tried her best to deal with the thoughts on her own. When they first started occurring, she could usually force herself to think about something else. If she tried really hard right at the beginning when the thought would come into her head, she could usually distract herself. However, if she left it for just a moment or more, then it would become very difficult to stop the bad thoughts and images. But then the thoughts started coming more frequently, and she couldn't distract herself. She tried other things—whistling or singing even—but she knew that if she did that in front of her family or at the store, someone would know something was wrong.

She thought a lot about what would happen if the cancer came back. Who would help her with all the daily tasks of running the house? This would send her into a panic. Tim was working really hard, and things were tough at work. There was no way he could take off time like he did after Emma was born and she had her surgery. Grace was at college, and she couldn't leave to help out. Juliet was just so busy with her sports; she was hardly ever at home, and Nancy couldn't expect her to give up the things she loved. It was just not fair.

One of the characteristics of intrusive thoughts and feelings is that they are not realistic or logical. They tend to spiral out of control until they lead you to a situation of pure panic. Nancy finds herself imagining how she will manage if the cancer comes back, and she goes on a thought journey that leads nowhere. It is quite common that these fears center on coping with everyday activities and responsibilities. For women, these thoughts often focus on how they would have to rely on other people to take care of daily matters. Perhaps these thoughts represent something symbolic about what women do to keep the lives of their family running smoothly, and having to rely on others for help is scary.

Nancy decided to join a support group for younger women with breast cancer. One of the nurses at the cancer center had suggested it, and Nancy thought perhaps it would be a good thing to do. The nurses had told her about it after her surgery and when she was having chemotherapy, but she just hadn't been ready or able to even think about it then. But now she was interested, and she went to her first meeting. She was very nervous at that first meeting, but the facilitator made her feel at ease. There were about eight women at the meeting, and Nancy thought she recognized one of them from the cancer center. She didn't say much at that first meeting; she just sat at the very edge of the circle of chairs and observed quietly. The guest speaker for the evening was a plastic surgeon, and he talked about breast reconstruction after breast cancer. Most of the women at the meeting seemed to have had this procedure.

"Oh, I just love that I don't have to wear a bra!" said one woman. "Having the other boob made smaller at the same time was the best thing I could have done." She proudly pulled her shirt tight over her chest, and the other women in the group chuckled in approval.

"I'm just happy I did it at the same time as my mastectomy," said another. "I just couldn't imagine having to go back for another surgery."

Nancy felt a little out of place and wondered if the other women or the surgeon could see that she was wearing a prosthesis. As she sat there, it began to physically irritate her. She tried to stop herself, but she felt her hand moving over to where the prosthesis sat under her bra. She tweaked the edge of it where it extended over the edge of the bra cup, and she felt it move against her skin and the scar, which was still sensitive two years after the surgery. She quickly moved her hand back to her lap and concentrated on what the plastic surgeon was telling them. She listened as he explained the different kinds of procedures, and as he talked, she thought about perhaps having this done for herself.

———⊗⊗⊗———

Support groups can be a good source of both information and support. There are different kinds of support groups, and it may take a while to find one that best meets your needs. Some support groups are disease specific (for example, a support group for women with breast cancer). Some are age specific, such as the group Nancy went to for young women with breast cancer. Some support groups encourage partners and family members to attend, while others are only for patients and survivors. There is usually a facilitator for the support group, and this person may be a professional, such as a social worker, or a layperson, such as another cancer survivor.

It is important to judge whether what is discussed at the support group meetings is valuable to you. Some support groups are focused on sharing information and have a guest speaker at each meeting. Other support groups are less focused, and those attending are free to talk about whatever they want. Sometimes these sorts of support groups turn into a gripe session about things that are not very constructive.

Research has shown that support groups that focus on problem solving or stress reduction are more effective in reducing anxiety and depression and in improving quality of life than groups with little focus. It is also important to keep in mind that the experiences of other survivors in a group may not necessarily translate to your experience. If you find that attending a support group makes you more worried or depressed, then perhaps you need to find another support group or to stop attending one entirely.

———⊗⊗⊗———

Nancy went home after the support group, her mind whirling with the new information, and the next morning she told Tim that she was thinking about having the surgery. Tim was not sure she should be having more surgery. He had gone back to work only after her chemotherapy was completed, and he was scared that he would need to take more time off work. His boss had been accommodating the first time, but he was not so sure he would be again. Things were more difficult at work. The publication company he worked for had started outsourcing a lot of the work to India, and Tim was terrified that his job would go offshore as well. He didn't tell Nancy most of this; she had enough to worry about. But he was worried, really worried. Nancy had told him repeatedly that she hated wearing the prosthesis. She said she felt lopsided if she didn't wear it, and it reminded her constantly of the breast cancer. He couldn't really argue with her, so she made plans to see the same plastic surgeon who had talked at the support group.

Having breast reconstruction is something that many women consider. It may be offered at the same time as the mastectomy, and many women prefer to do the two surgeries at once. It does increase the length of time the surgery takes, and not every cancer center may offer this as a choice. Other women choose to have reconstruction sometime after the initial mastectomy. There are a number of different procedures, including taking skin from the abdomen and using it to create the reconstructed breast. Other women have a saline or silicone implant. The choice of which kind of surgery to have may be dictated by factors such as body weight and availability of enough skin and fat to create a breast or to the skill and comfort of the surgeon who performs the reconstruction.

Nancy had the reconstructive surgery the summer before Juliet went to college, and once again her family had to pitch in and help with the household chores and taking care of Emma. Nancy couldn't lift anything for six weeks after the surgery, and little Emma would often cry to be picked up by her mommy. Nancy had the procedure where skin and fat are taken from the abdomen, and she was pleased to get rid of her pregnancy fat from her tummy. At first she couldn't even bear to look at her new breast. It looked so different from her other breast, and when she saw it in the mirror after her shower, it just made her want to cry. It was bigger and rounder, and the scar on her tummy was red and swollen and went from one hip to the other. The nurse at the plastic surgeon's office had warned her about this, but it still scared her to see these changes in her body. The nurse told her it would take months for the swelling to go down and for the scars to fade. But she was impatient. She just wanted to feel like she used to about her body and her life.

And she was still really anxious about the cancer coming back. A few months after her reconstructive surgery, she went to see the oncologist. He hesitated before examining her breasts, and she panicked immediately.

"What's the matter? What's wrong?" her voice crackled with fear.

"Don't worry. It's nothing," replied the oncologist. "I just didn't realize that you'd had reconstructive surgery. How is that working out for you?"

Nancy was not sure how to reply. On the one hand, she was happy she'd had it done, but on the other hand, she was not completely happy with the results. She tried to formulate her answer to his question, but she couldn't find the words.

"Many women find that the reconstructed breast is not quite what they had imagined it would be," continued the doctor as he gently examined her. "It can take a while before things settle, so just be patient."

Nancy felt the tears rush to her eyes. She was lying down, and they flowed out of the corners of her eyes and onto the paper covering the thin pillow.

"Hey, what's this?" The doctor quickly covered her chest with the crinkly paper gown and helped her into a sitting position.

"It's nothing, I just . . ." Nancy's voice cracked as she tried to get the words out and to stop crying at the same time.

"How about you get dressed and we can talk about this a bit more?" The doctor stood up, closed the curtain around the examination table, and then washed his hands as Nancy dressed quickly. She didn't know what she was going to say, but she was grateful that someone had recognized that she was not happy.

———

Many women are disappointed after they have reconstructive surgery. They may have unrealistic expectations, or they may just be frustrated when the healing period takes longer than they thought it would. The scars both on the breast and the abdomen are red for some months after the surgery, and it usually takes months for them to fade to pink and then eventually to a silvery white color. Some women, in particular African American women, may develop a thickening of the scar (called a keloid), and this can cause even more uneasiness for them.

———

Nancy and the doctor talked for quite a while. Well, she did most of the talking. She told him that she was not all that happy with the reconstruction, and for the first time she admitted to someone that she was having bad thoughts and was extremely anxious about the cancer coming back. The oncologist listened without saying much. He nodded his head every now and then, but once Nancy started talking, it was like a dam had burst. The doctor's face was creased in concentration as he listened to her long list of fears. Eventually she stopped, slightly out of breath and with a red face.

"I think this is more than I can handle," he suggested quietly. "I really think you should see our social worker."

Nancy drew in a breath and started to protest, but he interrupted her.

"Nancy, it's been some time since your diagnosis, and you have a lot of anxiety. I'm not saying there is something wrong with you, but most women are not suffering as much as you are at this point. That's all I'm saying. If you were still having pain at this point, I would send you to a pain specialist. Think of this as emotional pain. You need to see someone to help you. Okay?"

Nancy sat in the chair, her shoulders slumped in exhaustion. She knew he was right, but she just didn't think she was the type of person who would need this kind of help.

"I'm going to get the nurse to see if someone is available to meet with you now. You can wait here while we try to organize it. Okay?"

And with that, he left the room. Nancy remained in her chair, deep in thought. She didn't want to see the social worker now, but the oncologist had given her little choice. She was startled when there was a knock at the door and a woman entered the room. She was short with spiky red hair.

"Nancy? I'm the social worker. Barb Walker. Pleased to meet you."

She walked toward Nancy with her arm outstretched, her hand in position to shake Nancy's.

"Hello," replied Nancy, her hand lying in her lap.

Barb quickly drew her hand back and stopped where she was.

"Um, I was wondering if you would like to make an appointment to see me in the next couple of days. I can't spend much time with you today, but I have some openings in my schedule toward the end of the week."

Nancy opened her mouth to refuse, to make an excuse, but she thought better of it. Maybe this person could help. Maybe. She knew she needed help, so she agreed to see Barb later that week.

It can be very difficult to admit that you need help coping after cancer treatment. It is especially difficult months or even years after treatment, when you assume that you should be feeling like your old self. Many survivors believe they have to think and act and feel a certain way and not complain. They may even be given the message that they should just be happy to have survived when others have not.

Nancy didn't tell anyone that she was going to see the social worker. She was still not convinced that she would actually keep the appointment. A little voice in her head kept whispering that she didn't need any help. But every now and then she would look at Emma, and she would feel the tears come to her eyes as the familiar panic set in. Who would take care of Emma if the cancer came back? She imagined Emma's first day at school and then graduating from high school, and the thought of not being there for all those milestones made her breathing come faster and faster until she thought she would faint. So when Friday came, she told the girls she had to go to an appointment, and they were happy to take care of Emma for the afternoon.

She had to ask at the information desk at the cancer center where she could find the social worker. An elderly volunteer offered to escort her, and Nancy agreed, feeling as if she were the old person. The social work office was in the basement of the building, but it was nicely decorated with lots of green plants and bright yellow walls. Once again she was greeted by the social worker with an outstretched hand, and this time she took it and shook hands with the woman. They went into Barb's office, which contained a small desk and two large overstuffed armchairs. As Nancy sat down, she felt a sense of peace come over her. For the first time in a long time, she felt relaxed, which surprised her.

"So, Nancy . . . is it okay if I call you that?" the social worker started.

Nancy nodded.

"How can I help you?"

Nancy didn't know where to begin. She immediately felt the tears well up in her eyes, and she tried to blink them away. All this did was cause them to run down her face, and she angrily brushed them off with the backs of her hands. The social worker passed her a box of tissues and waited until Nancy found her voice.

"I don't know what's wrong with me," she began. Her voice sounded high to her own ears. "I just feel so bad about everything. I went and had the reconstructive surgery, and I don't like how that's turned out. I have these thoughts all the time, and they scare me. I think about getting sick again, and I just couldn't go through it again. I know I have so much to live for, but I just can't help it. I'm scared that the cancer is going to come back, and if it does . . ."

Nancy stopped talking, and her shoulders slumped. She stared at her hands in her lap and said nothing more. The social worker spoke in a soft voice:

"You sound really anxious. You're not alone in thinking and feeling this way. Many cancer survivors feel like this."

"I *hate* that word, 'survivor'!" Nancy spat out the words, her body suddenly upright in the chair. "What if the cancer comes back? Have I then failed at being a survivor? Why does everyone keep telling me I'm a survivor?"

The social worker sat back in her chair. She had heard these words, too.

"What would you call yourself, Nancy? How would you describe your place in the cancer journey right now?"

Nancy sat and thought about this for a moment. No one had ever challenged her on this topic before. She hadn't really told anyone that she felt so strongly about the word *survivor*, so she didn't have an easy answer to the question.

"I don't really know what to call myself. I haven't really thought about it. I just know that the word *survivor* makes me crazy. Do I have to call myself something? Can't I just be Nancy?"

"Of course you can be Nancy. You can be and call yourself anything you want. Some people say that a person with cancer is a survivor from the day they are diagnosed."

"Right!" Nancy snorted. "As if that counts. The day you are diagnosed, you become a patient, a victim of everything that is coming. And none of it is pretty!"

"Many would agree with you, and many would not. It's just words, Nancy. How about if we talk about how *you* feel now, at this point in your life, and see if we can figure out a way to help you help yourself?"

Nancy stared at the social worker for a minute. "How can I help myself? Don't you think I would already have done that if I could've?"

The social worker smiled gently. "Of course you would have. But sometimes a person just needs some outside help. When you're in a situation like you are, it's often hard to see what might help. So here's what I heard you say. You think a lot about the cancer coming back, and it scares you. You had reconstructive surgery, and you're not happy with the outcome. Am I on the right track here?"

Nancy nodded. When someone else said the words, it really didn't sound that bad. But in her head and heart, it felt bad, really bad.

"So where would you like to start first? What is your priority? The fear of the cancer coming back or how you feel about the reconstructive surgery?"

She made it sound so simple, Nancy thought. She had two choices to think about, and in an instant she knew that the fear of the cancer coming back was the most important to her.

"I think the cancer coming back."

"Okay, let's start!"

Finding and accepting help is a big hurdle to overcome. Many people resist seeking help because they think it means they are weak. We live in a society where there is a push-pull between the expectation of being so self-sufficient that you never ask for help and the helplessness of some people who seem unable to figure things out for themselves and constantly seek support and medication.

It can be difficult to identify exactly what is causing the emotional distress. Our feelings are just that—feelings—and it can be hard to put into words just what those feelings mean. A professional can help identify what it is that is bothering you or causing distress. And once you have that figured out, you can start working on a solution or resolution.

Barb the social worker explained to Nancy that fear of recurrence is a source of great anxiety for people after treatment is over. And women with young children seem to be the most anxious of all. Nancy seemed to relax as she heard these words. There was a reason! She was not some sort of freak or nutcase!

"So if this is 'normal' for women like you, what do you want to do about it? Here are some options. You can see a psychologist or psychiatrist and go on some antianxiety medication."

Nancy immediately shook her head. She hated taking pills, and she was afraid they would make her feel weird.

"Okay, so no pills." Barb smiled.

"There are some other things you can try. They are perhaps more challenging than just swallowing some pills once or twice a day. I'll present you with some of the strategies I've used with other clients, and you can pick and choose. One thing that people find helpful is to keep a diary in which you write down what you are thinking and what you are doing at the time to identify the patterns of negativity in your head."

Nancy interrupted her. "I have a little girl at home. I hardly have the time or energy to shower every day. I don't think having to write things down is going to do it for me."

"Okay. How about if we talk about refocusing your thoughts? You know, when you have a bad thought, for example, you feel a twinge of pain somewhere, and you immediately think it means the cancer is back. Refocusing means that you consciously stop that thought and replace it with something more logical and realistic."

"I don't know." Nancy seemed hesitant with this suggestion.

"Okay, I have more suggestions."

Keeping a diary and refocusing your thoughts are two strategies that can be helpful for people who find that they are having anxiety-provoking thoughts and feelings. It requires commitment and attention and may not be right for everyone. When keeping a diary, you would note the stressful event (such as having to go to the cancer center for follow-up care), and then you would note what it was about the event that made it stressful or anxiety provoking; what your physical and emotional reactions were to the event (for example, your heart beating faster); how intense these reactions were; how you handled the event; and what you would do differently the next time.

Connected with this is the strategy of refocusing your thoughts. So, for example, if you have to go to the cancer center for follow-up care, on the way there you may start thinking about bad news you might hear at your appointment. Like Nancy, your thoughts may shift to what would happen if the cancer is back. So your initial thought, "They are going to tell me the cancer is back," is replaced with a refocused thought, "I am just going for my regular follow-up appointment. I have not experienced any symptoms that suggest the cancer is back."

When you first start doing this, it may feel forced. But the more often you do it, the easier and more natural it will feel. The intent is not to make you happy all the time, but rather to help you avoid negative thinking and instead think more positively and realistically.

—⊗—

"So here are some other strategies that focus on relaxation for your body and that then help to relax your mind. Have you heard of progressive muscle relaxation? This is where you consciously relax the muscles in your body, starting at your feet and moving up to your head. Deep breathing is another technique that can help you relax. Does either of those sound interesting to you?"

Nancy thought about it for a moment and then shook her head. "I'm not sure I have the time. Emma, you know?"

Barb nodded in sympathy. "I remember when my son was a toddler. There was hardly time in the day to go to the washroom. But could you find fifteen minutes in your day, maybe two or three times a week? Perhaps when your baby is napping? It's better for you than folding laundry, although I know how important that can be!"

"Maybe I can try. I'm not sure. But I'll try."

—⊗—

Progressive muscle relaxation is a simple technique to learn and can help reduce stress and anxiety. Detailed instructions are provided in chapter 12. Deep breathing can also help with these relaxation exercises, or it can be done by itself. It may sound silly to have to learn how to breathe, but most of us don't do it properly. So a few minutes of instruction can start a lifetime of better breathing!

It is important to remember that no technique or intervention will help immediately. These things take time and patience and commitment. But they do not involve taking pills or experiencing side effects, and they may be a good place to start on your own.

—⊗—

Nancy went home feeling drained. She wanted to feel better, she really did. Perhaps she should try these relaxation exercises. Maybe they would help. When she got home, Juliet was playing with Emma in the kitchen. Emma had a bowl on the tray of her high chair, and she had been eating the scrapings of what looked like brownie batter. The kitchen smelled of chocolate and butter and sugar, and the little girl was covered in brown smudges. The look on her face when she saw her mother in the doorway made Nancy laugh.

"Mamma! Mamma!" she cried, "Mamma!" She held her arms above her head, her little face shining with happiness.

Nancy picked her up and, even though she was covered in batter, held the little girl close. When Emma wriggled to be let go, Nancy reluctantly released her, and the little girl toddled away, her excited giggles trailing behind her.

Nancy sat down in a kitchen chair, her body aching. It had been a long day, and there was still much to be done. An envelope on the kitchen counter attracted her attention. It was from the breast cancer support group. Nancy opened it as she chatted with Juliet about how her morning with Emma had gone. Inside the envelope was information about a special meeting of the support group, something to do with meditation. Nancy was about to throw the paper in the garbage when she stopped herself. Hadn't the social worker talked about meditation? Or maybe it was relaxation. Nancy looked at the invitation again. It was an evening about mindfulness meditation, and as she read the paragraph about it, Nancy found herself feeling interested. Maybe this would help! It said that mindfulness meditation could help women with breast cancer gain a sense of control over their lives by allowing them to live in the moment. That sounded very interesting, and Nancy got up to mark the date on the calendar. She was going to go to this session, and she hoped it would help.

Two weeks later, Nancy went to the support group meeting. She almost didn't go at the last minute, but the words of the social worker rang in her ears: What do you want to do about it? When she arrived at the support group, she was greeted warmly by a couple of the women who had been at the last session. This put her at ease, and she sat with them in the second row of chairs.

The speaker for the evening was a short man with a thin but muscular body. The facilitator of the group introduced him as Michael, but he interjected and told the audience of women that he preferred to be called Moo, his childhood nickname. The audience laughed, and he asked them to notice how their laughter had removed some of the natural nervousness they might have been feeling. Nancy felt herself being drawn into his voice, which was soft and almost singsong.

Michael, or Moo, explained that this evening would be an introduction to mindfulness meditation, an appetizer for the full six-course program that any of them could sign up for if they were interested. That night, he was going to tell them about this form of meditation and teach them the basics of meditation, breathing, and something he called the body scan technique. According to Moo, this form of meditation had been shown to help cancer patients reduce stress, promote relaxation, and even alleviate physical discomfort. One of the women sitting behind Nancy whispered rather loudly, "Sign me up, Scotty!" and the women around her had to struggle to muffle their laughter.

"So, shall we begin?" With these words, Moo began to teach.

Mindfulness-based stress reduction is a form of meditation and yoga that has been popularized by Jon Kabat-Zinn and his colleagues at the University of Massachusetts. It is usually taught as part of a six- or eight-week training program and has been used with people experiencing many different kinds of illness. It has been tested in clinical trials with breast and prostate cancer patients and has been shown to significantly improve mood and quality of life.

The focus of mindfulness meditation is on being present in the moment without getting distracted by memories of the past or anticipation about the future. The intention is not to bring about relaxation, but relaxation often does occur as a side effect. There are four kinds of mindfulness practice: awareness of sensation, sitting meditation, body scan, and mindful movement. A full description is presented in chapter 12.

Moo taught them how to breathe. He explained that although breathing is a natural and automatic action, most people do not breathe fully, using all of their lungs. People tend to use only the top part of their lungs, leaving out the bottom parts. By using the abdominal muscles to open the bottom part of the lungs as well, air is drawn into the entire capacity of both lungs, and this often elicits relaxation. In the beginning, there was some giggling among the women as they used their abdominal muscles to help draw air deep into their lungs. But they soon quieted down, and a feeling of calm seemed to enter the room. Moo talked in a quiet voice and asked the women to focus awareness on their bodies. He asked them to feel the fabric under their buttocks and legs. He then asked them to focus on their arms and notice where they were resting and what that felt like. Nancy followed his instructions, his voice drawing her attention to her body and then letting her just feel her body in silence. She had no idea how long this part took, but eventually Moo told them to bring their focus back to the room. Nancy opened her eyes, the light suddenly bright. She could not remember being told to close her eyes, but she had. The women shifted in their chairs, and one or two yawned loudly.

"Ladies, you have just experienced sitting meditation! And I bet you had no idea that was what you were doing! Congratulations! You are mindful meditators!"

Moo's enthusiasm was contagious, and the women laughed. One woman in the back row put up her hand and asked in a loud voice, "Is that it?"

"Yes, that's the beginning," Moo replied with a smile in his voice. "Pretty simple, huh? If you sign up for the rest of the course, you will find that what you have done here this evening forms the basis of your mindfulness practice."

"Where can we sign up?" was the response from more than one woman in the group. And Nancy was one of them.

The group facilitator then stood up and talked about where the rest of the sessions would be held. Nancy was a little concerned because they would all be during the evening. But then she decided that she had three competent baby sitters in the house, and she wanted to do this for herself. She really did. So she walked quickly to the table where the sign-up sheet was located and wrote her name and phone number down. The first session was the next week on a Monday evening.

There is some variation in how mindfulness meditation programs are taught. Most involve a weekly session of about an hour or more with homework sessions for the rest of the week. Some programs require participants to keep a diary of their practice. Participants are usually expected to do some form of meditation six days a week for fifteen to forty-five minutes.

Nancy has chosen this particular intervention to try to help herself, but there are others. Most are successful for many people. It is a matter of finding something that you can do regularly and to which you are willing to commit.

The weeks of the program flew by. Nancy found that she really looked forward to going to the Monday-evening sessions. There were about ten women from the support group who attended these sessions, and they had started going out for coffee after each session. It was nice to sit and chat with these women who had all been through the same thing. They didn't talk about cancer at all, but rather about their families and the daily challenges that confronted them. The group was about Nancy's age or a bit older, and the fact that she had a young daughter was a source of both amusement and horror for them. Nancy took their teasing in good humor. She showed them photos of the older girls with Emma, and everyone remarked on how lovely the three girls were. About four weeks into the program, one of the women tearfully told the group that her seventeen-year-old daughter was pregnant, and they all hugged her and offered any help they could. They lingered over coffee much longer that evening, and it was well after ten o'clock when Nancy eventually let herself into the house.

Tim was sleeping in front of the TV, and he woke with a start when he heard the door close behind her. "I'm sorry I woke you," she began, her voice low so as not to disturb the girls who were sleeping.

"That's okay. I must have nodded off. How was your group?"

"Great. I'm really glad I did this. We went out for coffee after, and Jan—you know, the woman whose husband was having an affair when she was having treatment? Well, anyway, she told us that her daughter is pregnant. The kid's only seventeen, and Jan is just devastated. Can you imagine if Juliet got pregnant?"

Tim was silent for a few minutes, and then he groaned. "That would definitely be a problem. But Emma would love being an aunt!"

Nancy tossed one of the throw pillows from the couch at him. "Don't joke about it, Tim! Honestly!"

But there was laughter in her voice, and when he stood up and pulled her into his arms, she put her arms around him. They stood there like that for a few minutes, and Nancy couldn't help but notice that in that moment her breath filled her lungs from top to bottom. She felt so peaceful, standing in the dark living room in the circle of her husband's arms, her daughters safe in their beds down the hall. For the first time in a very long time, she just knew it was going to be okay. Everything was going to be okay. Life was good.

· 3 ·

When Will I Be Happy Again?

*M*any cancer survivors find that, after all the activity and attention during the treatment phase, they are depressed. Often their family and friends don't understand why this is happening, and they tell the survivor to just be happy that they are alive. Robert is one such survivor. After almost a year of treatment for colon cancer, he is feeling really down and is not getting much support from his family, who just want the old husband and dad to be back.

The past two years have been a nightmare for Robert. It all started when he noticed some blood on the toilet tissue. The first time he saw it, he panicked, but then he thought about it a bit more and decided it was probably just hemorrhoids. It happened again the next day, and once again he told himself it was the hemorrhoids. And then it went away, and Robert just put it out of his mind. He was really busy at work. There had been cutbacks at the factory where he supervised the maintenance of the machinery, so he had even more to do. And his kids were at that stage where they needed a lot of attention. Billie was almost twelve years old and loved to play every sport under the sun, and Julie was fifteen and wanted to learn to drive. Most evenings were taken up with driving Billie to his games and either staying to watch or returning later to pick him up. There were weeks when he hardly saw his wife, Sue, and they joked ruefully that they were like ships in the night, passing each other in the dark.

And then it happened again—the blood on the toilet tissue. This time he couldn't explain it away. He had looked on the Internet for information about hemorrhoids, and he really didn't have any of the symptoms described. So what could it be? The article on the Internet said that bleeding could be a sign of something more serious, and that really bothered him. He tried talking to one of the dads at Billie's hockey game one Saturday afternoon. He knew the guy was a doctor, and when he saw him enter the rink he walked up to him.

"Hey, I'm Billie's dad. You know Billie—the big kid on left wing? Can I ask you something? It's a little embarrassing, but I know you're some kind of doctor and . . ."

The man cut him off. "Look, I don't mean to be rude or anything, but I just make it a rule that I don't give medical advice to anyone, anytime, anywhere. I just don't like to mix business with pleasure, and I'm here to watch my kid play hockey. Okay? No hard feelings, I hope."

And with that, he shook Robert's hand and walked off to join a group of parents who were sitting in the stands. Robert felt his face get red and hot. What a jerk! He went to get a cup of coffee just outside the rink, and when he came back, the game had started. He spent most of the game standing next to the boards, trying to ignore the group of parents in the stands.

He promised himself that if it happened again—the blood on the toilet tissue—he would do something about it. He just had this niggling feeling that something wasn't right. So he made an appointment to see old Doc Grant. Dr. Grant had looked after Billie and Julie since they were babies. He was an older man with thick white hair, and the kids seemed to like him. Sue, Robert's wife, usually took the kids to see him, and she said he was nice. Robert couldn't remember the last time he had seen a doctor. Maybe it was that year he hurt his back shoveling snow, or that time he sprained his ankle at work and needed a sick certificate to stay off his leg. He really couldn't remember.

He didn't want to worry Sue, so he called the doctor's office and made an appointment to see Dr. Grant at the end of the month. He was surprised it took so long to get an appointment, but then he put it out of his mind. The bleeding continued. In fact, it was getting worse. By the time the end of the month rolled around, there were drops of blood in the toilet after he had a bowel movement. He was really scared by the time he got to see Dr. Grant, who seemed surprised he had waited so long before seeing a doctor. He ordered some blood tests and made a referral to another doctor.

Within two weeks, Robert had the news, and it was not good. He had colon cancer and needed to have surgery immediately. His family was shocked and frightened. Sue hardly spoke to him after he told her. She was mad that he had waited so long, and also because he had not told her anything until he needed a ride to the hospital for one of his tests. The kids were just plain scared. Julie had cried for days after he told them, and Billie was just really quiet. He tried to reassure them, but he couldn't even convince himself. He was terrified.

It is quite common to avoid dealing with physical symptoms out of fear or wishful thinking. But ignoring something unusual will not make it go away. It is always better to deal with an unusual physical symptom promptly. Early diagnosis is very important when it comes to cancer. Over time, cancer tends to spread, and if it is caught early, the treatment is usually simpler. Robert is quite typical in thinking that the blood on the toilet tissue was hemorrhoids. That could be one of the causes. But bleeding from the rectum may also be a sign of colon or rectal cancer, so if it happens, it should be checked by a doctor.

Robert spent a week in the hospital after the surgery. He was in a lot of pain, and he fought with the nurses when they made him get out of bed. Sue and the kids came to visit him every day, but most of the time he was asleep. His recovery was slow once he got home. He had a large wound down the middle of his stomach, but the worst part by far was that he had a bag where his waste went. He could hardly bear to look at it. He had to lie on his back to sleep, and he had always slept on his tummy, so he hardly slept at all. He kept waiting for the bag to explode or leak. He really struggled to take care of it—there was a lot he had to learn with the bags and the sticky parts where the bag attached to his skin—but mostly he just hated its existence.

And then he had to have chemotherapy six weeks after the surgery. He was terrified at the prospect of being sick from the chemotherapy. He tried to tell his wife that he was thinking about not having chemo, and she just lost it with him. She cried and screamed and told him that if he didn't do everything he could to get better, she would take the kids and leave him alone to die. They didn't talk for three days after that, and he went for his chemo treatments with a heavy heart.

The nurses in the chemotherapy unit were great. They made a fuss over him every time he came in, and he was less anxious after they had taught him more about the drugs he was going to get. He trusted them. They were so professional and yet caring that he almost looked forward to each treatment. The treatments themselves were not that bad. He sat in a big comfortable chair as the drugs ran into his body. He had a special device implanted in his chest so the nurses didn't need to stick him with a needle for each treatment. They gave him some medication to prevent nausea which made him so sleepy that he mostly dozed during the treatments. He could watch TV or read while he was there, but he usually just slept or talked to the nurses. After two weeks, he noticed some tingling in his hands and feet, and the nurses reminded him that this was a side effect of one of the drugs. They encouraged him to report anything unusual, and he felt comforted that someone was listening to him. His hands and feet tingled most of the time now, and it was worse when he went outside in the cold. He often forgot to carry his gloves with him, and he suffered for his forgetfulness. His mouth was pretty sore, too. He had mouth ulcers, which made eating and drinking difficult. He avoided looking at the scale when the nurses weighed him before his treatments, but he could feel from his clothes that he had lost weight.

———

Colon cancer is usually treated with a combination of surgery, to remove the part of the colon where the cancer is, followed by chemotherapy. In order to allow the colon to heal after the surgery, a stoma, or opening, is created to allow waste (feces or stool) to leave the body. The stoma usually opens on the skin of the abdomen, and a bag is placed over it to collect the feces. Depending on where in the colon the cancer is, the waste that is collected may be more or less fluid. The stoma may be temporary or permanent.

Many people react with shock when they realize they have to live with a stoma. Feelings of disgust are also not uncommon. Like Robert, it may take some time to get used to the accommodations that need to be made in daily life to cope with the stoma and bag. Robert now has to sleep on his back, and this can be more difficult than at first thought. Some people have to change their eating habits and avoid foods that cause gas (like cauliflower, broccoli, and cabbage) because this may cause the ostomy bag to expand a lot. There are specially trained ostomy nurses who can help you learn more about your stoma and bag; these nurses are specialists and can give much-needed advice and support, especially in the early days of learning to live with the stoma.

Most people are very scared of having chemotherapy. They may have seen family members go through the treatment years before and are afraid of being sick. Things have improved over the years, and today powerful antinausea drugs are routinely given before chemotherapy to help with the nausea. However, chemotherapy does cause side effects, and despite the many good treatments for these side effects, some people still suffer. The chemotherapy used to treat colon cancer can also cause numbness and tingling in the hands and feet. This may make the usual activities of daily life challenging. For example, food preparation may be difficult, as the numbness may cause you to lose your grip on a plate or pan and drop it. It can also cause problems with walking and climbing stairs.

———

Things at home were pretty stressful. Sue did her best to be there for him, but she was doing all the work around the house, working her job as a teacher, and driving both kids to and from their many activities. She was not sleeping well. Robert could hear her getting up in the early hours of the morning, and she was short-tempered with everyone. The first few times Robert had chemo, he drove himself, but he found it too tiring to look for parking, so now he caught the bus. When the nurses heard this, they suggested that being in a crowded bus might expose him to too many germs, so they organized for a volunteer to pick him up at his house for his treatments and to take him home afterward. He was very grateful for everything they did for him.

The days and weeks passed slowly for Robert, but eventually he finished the treatments. The nurses had a little party for him on his last day. One of them baked a chocolate cake, and there were balloons and a card from all of them wishing him well. He didn't anticipate how emotional he would feel. They had taken such good care of him for almost six months, and now he would never see them again. He tried to hide the tears in his eyes, but Sandy, his favorite nurse, saw him wiping them away, and she came over and gave him a hug.

"It's okay, big guy," she whispered in his ear. "We all know you're not as tough as you make out. You'll be fine, just wait and see. Now get out of here! Go and live the rest of your life!"

Robert went home and opened the door to an empty house. Sue was at work, and the kids were at school. The silence was overwhelming in comparison to the chemotherapy unit he had just left. The sounds of the nurses' laughter echoed in his mind, and for a moment he wished he were back there, with the busyness and the beeping of the pumps and the phones ringing. His house, his home, felt empty, and he felt so alone in the place where he should have felt the most comfortable.

The end of treatment is a milestone for most people with cancer. The weeks and months of going to the hospital or cancer center are over, and many patients think they should celebrate this in some way. But often there is little to celebrate. At the end of chemotherapy, most people are at their weakest physically and often emotionally, too. This is a time when the side effects of chemotherapy are often at their worst.

Probably the most notable difference for patients is that they don't have to go for treatment anymore, and this leaves a lot of empty hours in the days and weeks ahead. As much as treatment can be difficult, there is also comfort in knowing that you are being well cared for. Seeing the nurses regularly makes many people feel safe. They know that they are being monitored and that the nurses will take care of any problems that occur. Many patients become very attached to the nurses in the chemo treatment area, and the end of treatment feels almost like a breakup of a relationship. Being at home alone after the intense period of treatment may feel lonely and strange, and most people are not prepared for this.

While going through active treatment, many patients find that the nurses and other health care providers become like a second family. But this is a special kind of family with no history, and the new relationships are intense and satisfying. The nurses had paid Robert a great deal of attention and had treated him like

he was special; at home, his wife was very busy and stressed due to her increased
responsibilities. Part of the transition out of active treatment means letting go of
the relationships that were formed as part of the treatment, and this can be very
challenging for some patients. There is even a term for this: deprofessionalizing,
which means reducing the amount of care-seeking behavior. But for most patients
it feels like loss or abandonment.

Over the next couple of months, Robert's body healed. The mouth ulcers got better, and he was able to eat and drink a little. The doctors had told him it would be another few months before he could go back to work, and he tried to make the most of his time away from the stresses of the factory. Some of the guys had come to see him while he was recovering from surgery, but the visit was awkward. They didn't have much to talk about other than work stuff, and they seemed uncomfortable to see him in his pajamas and housecoat. They did not visit again, but the factory manager sent a big fruit basket. It had arrived when his mouth ulcers were at their worst, and he couldn't even eat anything.

The days were long without anything to do. Sue and the kids were gone all day, and most evenings, after a quick supper, Sue took Billie to his games. Julie seemed more interested in her friends. She had her driver's license now, so she took his car and off she went. Robert tried to do more around the house, but that just seemed to make Sue angry. The second time he did the laundry, he put one of Billie's t-shirts in with Julie's white jeans and turned them pink. That was the last time he did the laundry.

Sue fell into bed exhausted every night. Within minutes, she was fast asleep, her face finally relaxed after the long day. They were hardly talking to each other, just brief questions and answers about things related to the kids or when she would be home. Robert stayed up later and later, the TV flickering in the dark of the family room. He dozed for a few minutes, and then his eyes would snap open. He tried to sleep in their bed but he couldn't. He tossed and turned, and then Sue would wake up.

"I have to get up in a few hours, and I can't sleep with you moving around like this. Honestly, you know what I have to do tomorrow!"

So he went back to the family room and whatever late-night comedian he could find on the TV. Most days he didn't shower until noon, and some days he didn't bother. No one seemed to notice if he shaved or not, either. He felt like a shadow in his own house, unnoticed by anyone and barely taking up space. His appetite was virtually nonexistent. He picked at some crackers during the day and drank the coffee that was left over from the pot Sue made each morning. It was lukewarm and bitter, but he hardly noticed.

*During the recovery period, things may not go back to normal, and there may
be some strain in relationships. For the months of active treatment, the partner of
the person with cancer is often left to deal with all the family and household responsibilities. As we see with Robert and Sue, she has taken on most of the household
chores and has continued to work and to care for the children and their daily activities. This can cause some resentment and then guilt. Sue has had to do the chores
because Robert has cancer, but her temper is strained, and she appears to be less than
supportive. Their kids have their usual routine, and Robert is the one who feels like
an outsider in his own home.*

Three months after his last chemo treatment, Robert had an appointment to see the surgeon. He had to repeat his name three times to the receptionist who seemed shocked at his appearance. "Robert? Is that you? You look
. . ." She hesitated, trying to find the right words. "Are you okay? You've lost
some weight. I guess the chemo . . ."

He wasn't listening and had turned to walk toward the chairs that lined
the waiting room. He sat in the corner, his body turned toward the window.
He stared out at the parking lot, deep in thought. Was any of this worth-
while? He thought by now that he would be feeling better, but if anything, he
was feeling worse. He hated the damned bag, and he hated feeling sick. He
felt worthless and useless. Tears welled up in his eyes, and he fought to keep
them from falling down his cheeks. Just then the receptionist called his name.
He stood up quickly with his back to her and brushed the tears from his face.

The surgeon seemed happy with Robert's progress. He checked his
abdomen and nodded as he inspected the scar and the placement of the bag.
"You eating okay? Any problems with the bag? Looks good to me. Hopefully
we can close off the ostomy in a while. Sound okay to you?"

He hardly waited for Robert to reply. He turned toward the sink and
washed his hands while Robert struggled for a moment to sit up and then
climbed off the examination table.

"You seem to be doing well. Any complaints?"

Robert opened his mouth to tell him how he really felt but then closed
it. The surgeon was getting up, his hand outstretched to shake Robert's.

"I'm fine. Glad to hear I can get rid of this bag. When did you say that
would happen?"

"Let me check your notes to see what the medical oncologist had to say.
My office will get back to you with a follow-up appointment. We'll discuss it
then." And then he was gone.

---

*Robert is clearly having some difficulties, but it seems no one is seeing this. He
is tearful and has lost a lot of weight. But the receptionist at the surgeon's office uses*

the chemotherapy as an excuse, and the surgeon hardly seems to see anything other than his ostomy bag and his surgical scar.

But Robert does not stop the surgeon from leaving the room. He remains silent other than to respond briefly to the surgeon's plans to remove the ostomy bag at some point in the future. Admittedly the surgeon didn't give Robert much of an opportunity to talk or ask questions. And Robert allowed him to do that. This is not uncommon. We know our health care providers are busy, so we don't demand their time to listen to our questions.

One solution to this problem is to make a list of questions that you want answered and take it with you to your medical appointment. Tell the doctor at the beginning of the appointment that you have questions you would like to ask, and use the list as a prompt. Don't leave the questions for the very end of the appointment without warning the physician that you want answers. If this doesn't work, make an appointment specifically to ask the questions. It might be useful to ask for the doctor's last appointment of the day, when he or she is not rushed to see the people waiting in the crowded waiting room.

Robert returned home from the appointment feeling disappointed, even though the news that the bag was going to be removed was good. These last months had been difficult, and he just didn't know what to do. The bag really did irritate him. He was constantly scared it was going to burst, and just looking at it made him feel sick to his stomach. But he was also so tired, and he just wanted to feel like his old self again. Nothing seemed to interest him anymore, and he felt useless. The kids didn't seem to need him anymore, and Sue was distant. Now that he thought about it, nothing gave him any pleasure. He hadn't watched any of the TV shows he used to like, and late at night, he didn't really watch the TV. He just liked the noise in the background. The guys at work had not visited again, and he wondered if they even remembered that he used to be one of them. For a few moments, the thought flickered through his head: What if he wasn't around? Would anyone really care? He felt the tears flood his eyes as he thought about what would happen to his family if he wasn't around anymore. The kids were self-sufficient now. Julie could drive and would soon go off to college. Billie was growing up too, and in just a few years he would be driving as well. Sue seemed to be managing all the household things, and she never asked for his opinion or discussed anything with him anymore. So what did they need him around for?

His thoughts were interrupted by Sue, who had come home early. She took her time putting away the groceries she had picked up, and Robert didn't get up to help her. He was tired most of the time and had stopped helping with the household stuff. And today he simply couldn't face her. He just wanted to be alone in the darkening room. He wondered if she would ask him about his doctor's visit that afternoon, but then he couldn't remember if she even knew he was going to the doctor. What had happened to them? They used to be so close, but now they were like roommates who were not even friends. He couldn't remember the last time they had laughed together. And they certainly hadn't made love for many months. Just thinking about all this made him feel even lonelier, and he wanted to curl up into a little ball. He decided to go and lie down in bed, even though it was not yet time for dinner. He tried to walk quietly so Sue would not notice him. But she heard his footstep on the bottom stair, the one that always alerted them when the kids came home after their curfew.

"Robert? Is that you? What are you doing?"

"Um, I'm just going to get something." Even to his own ears his voice sounded funny. It was high and squeaky as if his words were being squeezed out of a tight hole.

"What's wrong? What's the matter? Has something happened?" Sue's voice grew louder as she left the kitchen and came toward him. As she entered the hallway, she switched on the overhead light, and the small space was suddenly as bright as daylight. He tried to move away so she wouldn't be able to see his face, but it was as if he was rooted to the step. He felt the tears on his cheeks but didn't even have the will to wipe them away.

"Robert! Why are you crying? What happened? What is it?" Her voice echoed her rising panic. She took in the sight of him, his tears running down his face, his grip on the railing turning his knuckles white.

"I don't know!" he sobbed, any attempt at control long gone. "I don't know what's wrong. I just want . . . I just think you'd be better off without me!"

Sue stopped in her tracks, her face frozen in shock. "What? What are you saying?"

Robert sat down on the bottom step. His shoulders sagged, and he stared at his feet. "I'm of no use, Sue. Just look at me. I'm a useless piece of rubbish. I haven't been a good husband or father in the last few months. You'd be better off without me. At least you'd get the insurance money."

Sue was speechless for a moment; she stood looking down at him, her face white and pinched. "Robert! Just stop it! Stop talking nonsense! Just you stop it right now!" Her voice was shrill and her hands fluttered in front of her face. For a second she put her hands over her ears, as if trying to block out the sound of his voice. But he was not talking any more. He was just sitting on the stairs, his face in his hands, crying quietly.

—◦◦◦—

Robert has some of the classic signs of depression, including sadness, lack of pleasure in life (anhedonia), hopelessness and helplessness, low self-esteem and low self-worth, feelings of guilt, and suicidal thoughts. Another important sign of depression is difficulty sleeping. These are not unusual in the cancer survivor, and some studies estimate that up to 25 percent of people with cancer experience depression. Age, gender, type and stage of cancer, and the presence of social support all affect how often depression occurs, and depression can be experienced anywhere in the cancer journey, from diagnosis to the end of life.

And depression can happen after treatment is over. Given what we know about all the attention and busyness involved in the fight for survival during cancer treatment, it is easy to see how people can get depressed when the treatment is over.

The role of the cancer patient is quite clearly defined: you have to fight the cancer with all your energy, and you give yourself over to being taken care of by efficient and caring health care providers. Then you get through with the treatment, and then . . . well, then what? People around you may assume that after active treatment is over, you go right back to being the person you were before. But how can you be the same as you were before? You may assume that you have to get back to the old you, and you may have an unrealistic timetable for doing that.

We know that depression can profoundly affect the quality of life of the cancer survivor. And it can also increase the risk of relapse after treatment. Some studies suggest that depression can even affect survival. These are serious consequences, so depression should be identified early and treated. Some cancer care providers routinely ask patients and survivors if they are feeling depressed or are showing other signs of distress (depression is a sign of emotional distress). They may use screening tools (a brief questionnaire, for example) at every visit or ask the person if he or she is feeling sad or isn't sleeping well. Others don't ask about this and may even assume that depression is a normal part of the cancer experience.

—⊙∞⊙—

Sue sat down on the stairs next to her husband and for the first time in many months put her arms around him and let her head rest next to his. It felt strange to both of them for the first few moments, but then Robert relaxed into the circle of her arms and felt a wave of warmth flow through and over him. They sat there for a while, neither of them speaking. Robert had stopped crying, but every now and then he let out a huge sigh. Sue said nothing and continued to hold him in her arms. Eventually her arm started to cramp, and as she moved it the spell broke. Robert started to stand up, straightening his back and legs slowly. He hesitated for a moment as if he didn't know where to go, and Sue stopped him from walking away.

"Rob, you need to do something about this. You can't go on like this."

He looked at her, his face now calm. "What am I supposed to do? You know I'm right. The only thing that could help me is if I could turn back the clock and none of this happened."

"Well, you can't do that. We just have to deal with what has happened. When did you last see any of your doctors?"

His face colored slightly as he admitted that he had seen the surgeon just that afternoon.

"What? Why didn't you tell me? For goodness sake, Robert! I honestly don't know what to do with you! Do you not think that maybe, just maybe, I would want to come with you to these appointments? Why do you shut me out like this, Robert? Why?"

Robert didn't have an answer for the last part. As he thought about it, he realized that he had shut her out. He had kept her out of his life as he tried to cope with his treatment and the aftereffects. He was not sure why he had done this, but it was another part of his life that he wished he could turn the clock back on.

"The doctor said today that he was going to take away the bag. It means another surgery, I guess, and he was going to check with the oncologist."

"That's great!" Sue responded. "That's really great. Not the surgery part, I mean. But it'll make a difference for you without the bag, won't it?"

They had never really talked about his ostomy bag in all the months since his original surgery. It felt odd to be talking about it now, but Sue seemed to be grabbing on to this as a lifeline. He grunted in response to her excitement, and she carried on, her face animated and her words rushing out of her mouth in a tumble.

"Do you think you'll be able to go back to work, when the bag is gone, I mean? Not that I want you to go back to work. You should only do that when you're ready. But maybe that's what you've been waiting for. Maybe that's what's been holding you back from getting completely better, I mean."

Robert was not sure what to say. He had never told her how much the ostomy bag bothered him. But he was not sure that getting rid of it was going to solve all of his problems. In his heart of hearts he knew that what he was feeling and thinking wasn't normal. But he didn't know what to do about it, and he surely didn't have the energy to figure it out. Maybe he should talk to one of the nurses in the chemotherapy unit. Yes, that was it! He would call them in the morning. Or, even better, he would go there and see if they noticed anything. He managed a small smile, just at the corners of his mouth, and he could see that Sue responded to this slight movement with a big smile of her own.

It is not easy to admit that you are depressed. Sometimes it's even harder to admit it to someone you love. A big part of depression may be your inability to get motivated enough to ask for help or to describe how you are feeling.

People cope in different ways, and how you cope in general may predict your likelihood of becoming depressed. For example, if you tend to be less optimistic in your overall outlook, you may be more likely to become depressed after cancer treatment is over. If you use denial as a coping mechanism, you are also more likely to become depressed after treatment. People who have any kind of difficulty with everyday activities are also more likely to be depressed after treatment. And if you have problems with depression before cancer treatment, you are even more likely to be depressed afterward.

The next morning, Robert was up early. He dressed quickly after his shower and was in the kitchen making the coffee when Sue stumbled in, her hair standing up in clumps and her face creased from the pillow. She squinted at him from behind her bangs and nodded in appreciation when she saw that the coffee was almost ready.

"Why are you up so early?" she asked.

"I think I'm going to go to the hospital, just to pop in on the nurses in the chemo unit."

"Oh, okay. Is there anything the matter? Why do you need to see them? Do you want me to come with you?"

He could see that she was trying to be helpful, and he felt grateful for this, even though it was too little, too late. "That's okay. They don't know I'm coming. I'll just pop in before they get busy."

Her attention had already wavered, and she was now standing in front of the refrigerator, scanning the shelves for something to take with her for lunch. Robert finished his coffee, considered eating a bowl of cereal, and then decided he would pick up some muffins for the nurses on his way to the hospital. Sue had gone upstairs to shower and dress. He left the house quietly, started the car, and then backed down the drive and into traffic. It was not yet eight o'clock, and there were few cars on the streets. He listened to the radio and almost forgot to pull into the drive-through at Dunkin' Donuts to buy the muffins.

After a brief stop to buy a dozen fresh muffins, he was on his way and had no difficulty finding a parking spot just a block away from the doors of the hospital. The hallways were already busy, and Robert hardly noticed the crush of medical students and residents who rushed past him on the way to their different areas. He was a little out of breath from the short walk, but he blamed this on the box of muffins he was carrying. The chemo unit was just beginning to wake up when he pushed his way through the double doors. The first person to greet him was Jeannie, the receptionist.

"Hey, Robert! Nice to see you. Did you have an appointment today? I don't see your name on the list."

"No, I'm just here to give the girls a treat. Here, have one yourself!" He offered the box to Jeannie, and she waved him away with an apologetic smile.

"I can't touch those things, much as I love them. They just don't agree with my hips and butt!" She laughed as she pushed her chair back, exaggerating her need to be as far away from the muffins as possible. One of the nurses popped her head around the corner, looking to see which of her patients was there early.

"Robert! You're back! Nothing wrong, I hope. What can we do for you?"

"Hi, Judy. I just came by to bring you girls a treat. I wanted to say . . ." And to his embarrassment, he started to cry. He stood in front of the desk, holding the box of muffins, with tears pouring down his face. There was nothing he could do to stop them. Judy gestured for him to come through the doors at the side of the reception desk. He had walked through those doors so many times over the past months, and never once had he done so with tears running all over his face. He was still holding the muffins as Judy ushered him quickly into one of the private rooms where patients could lie on a gurney to have their chemotherapy. She closed the door firmly behind her and motioned him into the chair.

"What's going on, big guy?" Her voice was soft even though she used a pet name for him. He was a large man, almost six feet, three inches, but at that moment he felt like a very little boy.

"I don't know. I've been like this a lot lately. I can't seem to help myself. I just seem to cry for no reason." His voice came out in gulps as he removed one hand from the box of muffins and tried to wipe his face.

"It sounds to me like you need to talk to someone. Let me see if the social worker is around. It's a bit early, but maybe she's here." Judy already had the telephone in her hand and had started to punch in the numbers.

"No, wait!" Robert almost shouted. "I don't want to see the stupid social worker! I shouldn't have said anything! Just leave it alone, please, Judy!"

Judy stopped what she was doing and gave him a stern look. He remembered that look from once before when he hadn't told her how bad his mouth sores were and she had been mad at him.

"Robert! Not one more word. If you don't want to see the social worker, that's okay. But you have to see someone. I've seen this before, and it won't go away or get better on its own. So who's it going to be? The social worker or the psychiatrist? Your choice, big guy. But you have to see someone."

It is often very difficult to ask for help or to even accept help when it is offered. Robert was perhaps seeking help by going to visit the nurses at the hospital where he had received his chemotherapy. He knew that they would help him, and so he went there.

The nurse realized that emotional distress, which for Robert manifested as depression, is common in cancer patients and survivors, and she insisted that he see someone, a social worker or a psychiatrist, for help.

———◆———

Robert saw the psychiatrist the next week. His offices were in the same hospital where Robert had had his cancer surgery. He was not sure why he chose the psychiatrist over the social worker, but he was nervous when he entered the waiting room of the doctor's office. It was like all the other waiting rooms in the hospital—with straight-backed chairs placed around the edge of the room, a reception desk in the center of one wall, and piles of old magazines on small tables in the corners. He told the receptionist his name and then sat down along the wall facing the door. He was twenty minutes early, and while he waited, he remained alone. The receptionist was busy typing on her keyboard and answering the phone; she didn't look up or engage him in conversation.

At just one minute past his scheduled appointment time, the receptionist called his name. He was still the only person in the waiting room. He followed her through a door and into an office. The psychiatrist was sitting behind a large wooden desk. He glanced up from his computer when Robert entered the room and motioned for him to sit in one of the three chairs or a low couch placed together at the side of the room.

"The shrink's couch!" thought Robert, "It's exactly like in the movies!"

He deliberately chose one of the chairs and sat down carefully, his knees together and his hands clasped tightly on top of them.

"Good morning, er, Robert, is it?" the psychiatrist stood up from behind his desk and came toward Robert, his hand extended.

"Yes, Robert Jamieson." Robert tried to stand to shake the doctor's hand, but the chair was low and soft and he had some difficulty extricating himself.

"Sit, sit," the man repeated as he sat down on one of the other chairs which seemed firmer. "I'm Dr. Marks. How can I help you?"

Robert opened his mouth, but no words came out. He closed it and tried again. Still nothing. He felt really stupid, sitting there with his mouth opening and closing like a fish.

"Maybe I can help. The note I received from the nurse said that you were feeling depressed. Do you agree with that?"

Robert nodded, his throat tight and dry. He felt the prick of tears behind his eyes and fought them with all his power. He did not want to cry in front of this man! He would not! But then, as if by magic, his throat opened and a torrent of words rushed out. He told the psychiatrist everything, his words tumbling over each other, silent tears once again washing over his face.

Dr. Marks listened, nodding his head occasionally, but all the time keeping his eyes on Robert's face. When Robert was finished, about ten minutes had passed. The psychiatrist asked permission to speak. Robert was drained and nodded his assent. The psychiatrist told him that he had all the signs of something called posttraumatic stress disorder (PTSD).

PTSD? Robert was shocked. He knew that this was something that soldiers got from being in wars. But he had cancer! How could he possibly have this other thing? The psychiatrist explained it carefully, and as he talked, Robert found himself agreeing with most of what he was saying. But what could be done about it?

———

Some cancer survivors have the typical signs of posttraumatic stress disorder, usually seen in those who have experienced some kind of traumatic event. The symptoms of this for people with cancer include reliving certain treatments, experiencing difficulties getting to sleep and staying asleep, nightmares, and difficulties resuming normal relationships. This can be treated with counseling and also with antidepressant medication. If it is not treated, the person may experience significant challenges in making the transition from cancer patient to cancer survivor.

———

The psychiatrist suggested that Robert take medication in combination with regular visits for counseling. He also suggested that Robert get into the habit of doing some regular exercise. Robert was a bit surprised at this last piece of information. What did exercise have to do with anything? Dr. Marks saw the look on his face.

"Exercise has been shown to help with depression. Yes, I know, it seems as if exercise is the answer to everything these days, but it really does seem to help. Just give it a try and see what you think. Just a daily walk for thirty minutes or so will be fine. Can you manage that?"

Robert felt himself bristle. He used to play a mean game of hockey just a couple of years ago! And then he smiled when he realized that the doctor was trying to use humor to motivate him. Dr. Marks went to his desk and scribbled something on a small piece of paper. He handed it over to Robert, who stuffed it in his pocket without looking at it.

"That's a prescription for an antidepressant. It's what we call an SSRI. Take it as directed, and you'll start to see an improvement in your mood in about four to six weeks. I want to see you again in about two weeks, and then I will increase the dose. I like to start low and slow. You may notice some mild side effects—sleepiness perhaps, or changes in appetite. These will go away over time. Make an appointment with Beverly on your way out, and I'll see you in two weeks."

Robert stood up carefully. That was it? He shook the doctor's hand and looked for the door. It was right behind him, and he left the office without saying anything. The receptionist, Beverly, was on the phone, and she held up her hand with one finger in the air which Robert interpreted as a sign telling him to wait. She finished her conversation quickly and motioned him to come closer.

"When does Dr. Marks want to see you again?"

"Umm, he said in three weeks' time."

"Okay, then. How about the same time in exactly three weeks?" She was busy typing something into her computer and didn't look up.

Robert was still standing in front of her desk, and then he realized that he hadn't answered her. "Oh, sure. That would be fine."

She handed him a card with the doctor's name and office address on one side and his appointment date and time on the other. He took it and left without another word. He went straight to the drugstore and waited while the pharmacist filled the prescription. When the pharmacist called his name, he hurried over to the counter.

"Mr. Jamieson, have you ever taken this medication before?"

Robert shook his head.

"Well, then, let me tell you about the side effects."

"No thanks. I'm in a bit of a hurry, and anyway the doctor told me about them. Can I just go now, please?" He handed over his credit card, signed the slip of paper, and walked quickly to his car. He went back to his empty house, poured a glass of water, and swallowed the first pill. As it went down his throat, he said a silent prayer that it would work, that he would feel better, and that he could just get on with his life.

There are different classes of antidepressant drugs; they all act in slightly different pathways in the brain. Although there is little research on the effectiveness of these drugs in cancer patients specifically, there is good evidence that they are helpful in healthy adults with depression. The choice of drug is usually made on the basis of potential side effects, and the drugs in the SSRI (selective serotonin reuptake inhibitor) class seem to have the fewest side effects.

Cognitive behavioral therapy (a kind of talk therapy) has been shown to be effective in treating depression, and many psychiatrists offer a combination of medication and counseling. Some people find support groups helpful. There is increasing evidence that exercise can have a beneficial effect on mood, but this has not been tested extensively in people with cancer.

The days went by slowly until his next appointment with the psychiatrist. Nothing seemed different. He still struggled to get a decent night's sleep, and he thought about the cancer a lot. He was also waiting to hear from the surgeon about removing the bag and reconnecting his colon, and he spent most days in the house, waiting for the phone to ring with news about that. Sue had seemed relieved when he told her he was taking the pills, and she offered to come with him to his next visit with the psychiatrist. He was not sure what purpose that would serve, so he ignored her.

The morning he was scheduled to see Dr. Marks, he woke up later than usual and had to rush to get ready. Sue had already left for work, and the kids were either sleeping or at school. He brushed his teeth, showered hurriedly, and decided not to shave. The traffic was heavy, and he cursed as he waited to back out of the driveway, a stream of cars passing by on the busy street. He made it to the hospital with just minutes to spare and walked quickly to the psychiatrist's office. He smiled at the receptionist, recalling that her name was Beverly, and she told him to go directly in. Dr. Marks was once again at his desk. He looked up as Robert entered the room and smiled.

"How are you, Robert?"

"A little bit better, I think." As the words left his mouth, Robert realized that they were true. He did feel a bit better. But the change was so subtle that he didn't realize it until he said it. "I slept better last night than I have in ages. I didn't get up once! That has not happened since, well, since before the surgery. Could the pills be working that quickly? You said . . ."

Dr. Marks nodded as he walked over to the arrangement of chairs. Robert and the doctor sat down at the same time, both of them in the chairs they had sat in previously.

"Yes, the pills could be working this quickly. It's perhaps a little unusual, but good news is always good, right? What else is going on with you? Have you managed to get in some exercise?"

Robert colored slightly. He had tried to go for a walk soon after he saw Dr. Marks, but he didn't enjoy walking by himself. Truth be told, he found it quite boring. He told Dr. Marks this and also that he had been waiting around the house most of the day to hear from the surgeon. They talked about this for a while, and Robert admitted that his biggest problem was the colostomy bag. He described how it disgusted him and how eager he was to have his colon reconnected so that he didn't have to have the bag anymore. Once again, Dr. Marks listened as Robert poured out his heart. He told the psychiatrist things he had never said out loud before, not to Sue or even to himself. He described how disgusted he felt with how he looked and how he had avoided Sue and any chance of her touching him. He talked about how useless he felt as a man and as a father. It felt good to get it off his chest, and as he talked he realized he had bottled up a lot inside himself for a long time. Dr. Marks didn't say anything as the words and feelings flowed. He sat and nodded, and sat some more. After about fifteen minutes, Robert ran out of words. He sat back in his chair, exhausted and yet somehow relieved at the same time. It felt good to get all of those emotions out! If this is what counseling was about, then he thought it was a really good idea!

But then Dr. Marks took over. When Robert stopped talking, he started to ask questions, and Robert answered as best he could. Some of the questions were difficult: What had he done to try to resolve these feelings? Well, not much, it turns out. Why was that? How did he usually deal with adversity? Robert wasn't the kind of person to think about things like this. He came from a family where you kept your feelings hidden or else you got whipped for being a baby. He had never seen his parents really talk to each other. His dad mostly yelled, and his mother bit her lip and did what he wanted. It was like a light going on in his head as he saw the patterns emerge from answering Dr. Marks' questions.

Very soon, too soon, an hour had passed, and Dr. Marks ended their session. He told Robert to think about what they had discussed over the next two weeks, after which they would meet again. He encouraged Robert to try to get out for some exercise even though he thought it was boring. He also suggested that, instead of waiting passively for the surgeon's office to call, perhaps Robert should contact them and ask for information about future surgery.

Robert seems to be making some progress. The pills may have begun to improve his mood, and this may also have played a role in his ability to think more clearly and open up to the psychiatrist about his depression. This treatment combination—medication plus counseling—can be very effective in treating depression.

Many people are a little afraid of counseling. They assume they are going to have to tell all their deep, dark secrets. But often counseling shows us how our thoughts and feelings interact with our behavior. It can be very useful in changing how we think about events and for finding a more positive outlook on life or dealing with difficult situations. It has been shown to be very effective in treating depression, insomnia, and different kinds of anxiety disorders.

Robert went home with a plan—he was going to call the surgeon's office immediately and get an answer! He felt so much better already.

· 4 ·

What Will Everyone Say?

$\mathscr{M}$any cancer survivors want to go back to work after treatment, but this is not always easy. Steve is a construction worker, and he went back to work six weeks after having surgery for prostate cancer. He finds that he is still having some side effects of the surgery, and he struggles to keep up with his coworkers on the job site.

Steve hardly knew what hit him. At forty-eight years of age, he prided himself on being healthy. He hadn't needed to see a doctor for years, and he managed to keep up with the younger guys at work with no problem. His work in construction kept him fit, and he enjoyed playing baseball in a community league with guys almost twenty years young than himself. It was at a baseball game on a sunny spring Sunday that he felt a searing pain in his left knee. The pain almost took his breath away, and he hobbled in from the outfield to his car. He sat there for a while, the pain less severe, watching the guys finish the game. His knee felt hot to the touch, and it hurt if he moved at all. But he gritted his teeth and drove home, with beads of sweat on his brow and his jaw clenched.

Bonnie, his wife of twenty-five years, had to hide a grin when she saw him inching up the path from the garage. She had warned him over and over that he was going to get hurt one day. He wasn't as young as the rest of the guys, but he played as if he was a teenager. She tried her best not to say "I told you so" and helped him into a chair in front of the TV. She gave him some anti-inflammatory medication and a big glass of ice water and went back to the kitchen where she was making muffins for the kids to take to school on Monday.

Steve had hardly been sick in all their years together. She was a little surprised at how wimpy he was. He sat in the chair and moaned quietly every time he shifted.

45

"Can I get you anything?" she called out from the kitchen.

"No, I'm fine. I can manage," was his reply, his voice high pitched and obviously attention seeking.

"You'd better get that checked out. Do you want to go to the urgent care place?"

"No, I don't think so. Maybe it'll be better tomorrow."

"Well, I think you should call Dr. Browning first thing in the morning. You're working the late shift this week, right? Maybe he can see you before you go to work."

"Um, okay. Let's see how I feel in the morning. Hey, honey, could I get a beer?"

Bonnie smiled as she went to the refrigerator, picked up an ice-cold can of beer, and took it to him. He did look pathetic sitting in that chair. His foot was on a stool, and his knee looked swollen. Bonnie was a nurse, and even though she took care of kids at the Children's Hospital rather than adults, she had to sympathize with her husband. For the rest of the day, she fussed around him, bringing him a sandwich for dinner and helping him into the shower before bed. She tucked a pillow under his knee when he finally settled down for the night and made sure he took some more anti-inflammatories before he went to sleep.

The next morning, she left the house at her usual time, long before anyone else was awake. She called Steve on her break, and he told her he had called Dr. Browning and had an appointment at eleven o'clock.

"Let me know what he says," she instructed her husband. "Maybe you should call in sick to work, too. You haven't had a sick day in ages, and you really shouldn't be climbing scaffolding and carrying heavy stuff."

It is not unusual for men to have little if any contact with health care providers unless they injure themselves or are acutely ill. This may be due to socialization; men are not supposed to show signs of weakness, and seeking medical help could be perceived as a weakness. Women, on the other hand, are encouraged to seek regular medical care, usually because women are expected to seek attention for reproductive health care issues.

Steve agreed to call in to work and tell them he was too sick to come in for his shift later that afternoon. He managed to get dressed, pulling on a pair of shorts instead of jeans. His knee was not as swollen anymore but it still hurt, mostly when he put his full weight on it. He was glad he drove an automatic and didn't have to shift gears with his leg. He climbed the three stairs into the old house where Dr. Browning had his offices and was happy to sit down in the waiting room. He was a few minutes early for his appointment, and he looked around the room. He was the only man there. There were three young moms with their kids who were playing with the toys in the corner. One little girl looked like she had a fever, and she sat in her mom's lap, her face flushed and her body listless.

He was called in to see the doctor about ten minutes later. Dr. Browning was a cheerful if slightly harried man in his late sixties. He seemed surprised to see Steve.

"What brings you in today, Steve?"

"It's my knee. I was playing baseball yesterday, and it just went."

Dr. Browning motioned for Steve to sit on the examination table. He felt his knee, asked him to flex and extend it, and made some notes on the chart.

"Let's see how it goes over the next week or so. If it improves, you're in the clear. If not, then I'll send you to see someone." The doctor paged through Steve's chart. "When last did you have a checkup? It looks like it's been a really long time."

Steve cleared his throat. "I guess not since, well, I can't really remember."

"Well, you need one. You're not a young man anymore. I'll tell you what. I'm going to send you for some blood work, and you come back to see me next week. Jenny at the desk will take you to the lab and take your blood. I'll check on the knee when I see you again, and also check out the rest of you. Make an appointment at reception on your way out. See you next week."

Dr. Browning made some check marks on a small notepad and then tore off the sheet and handed it to Steve. Steve walked gingerly out of the exam room and back into the waiting room. He made an appointment for the next week, and Jenny took him to a small room down the hall where she expertly drew a couple of test tubes full of his blood.

———

The U.S. Preventive Services Task Force recommends the following annually for men aged forty to fifty years: measurement of blood pressure, height, and weight, and dental health screening. It also recommends that men in this age group have their cholesterol checked every five years.

———

Steve slowly got better. He went back to work two days later, and though his knee ached, he managed to do what he needed to on the construction site. He actually felt better by the end of the week and thought about canceling his appointment with Dr. Browning. But he had told Bonnie that the doctor wanted him to have a checkup, and she would be mad if he didn't go.

The following Monday, he once again went to the doctor's office. He had to get into one of those crinkly paper gowns he didn't like, and he was even less impressed when the doctor insisted on doing a rectal exam. He was glad his face was turned toward the wall because he could feel himself getting red. But it took just a few seconds and it was over. The doctor took his blood pressure and listened to his chest. He spoke to Steve as he washed his hands. "I'd like to go over the results of your blood tests with you. Get dressed, and I'll be back in a few minutes."

In a little bit, Dr. Browning returned, his attention focused on a piece of paper in his hand. "Hmm," he began. "So everything looks okay except for your PSA. It's a little on the high side for someone your age. Your prostate felt okay on examination, but I would like you to see a urologist just to be sure. I'll send off that referral and you'll get a call from his office. Any questions?"

Screening for prostate cancer using the PSA test is very controversial. Recent recommendations from a number of medical bodies recommend that men talk to their physicians about the pros and cons of having the test. It should not be done routinely, and certainly not without discussing it with the patient.

Steve didn't know what to think. He was not sure what all of this meant, so he kept quiet about it. Three days later he received a call from a Dr. Paul's office. They had an opening the next day and wanted Steve to come in. He was still working the late shift, so he had the time. He was just not sure what all this was about. But he went. The doctor, a urologist, was a younger man. He was rather abrupt and didn't explain much.

"It seems your PSA is up. That's not usual for a man your age. You need a biopsy. We can do that now or you'll have to wait. It's best to get it over with."

Steve agreed and had the biopsy. It hurt, and it was really embarrassing to be lying there with this probe up his rear end, but it was over in a few minutes. He was told to expect some bleeding, and off he went. Three days later, there was a message on his voice mail when he got home from work: the urologist needed to talk to him. Steve had a sinking feeling in the pit of his stomach, but he didn't tell Bonnie what had happened. The next morning he called the urologist's office, and the receptionist told him that he needed to see the doctor and that he should bring his wife with him. She made an appointment for him for two days later at the end of the day.

Now Steve had to tell Bonnie, and as he expected, she was mad at him for not telling her anything that had gone on. She went with him to the appointment, and in just a few moments their life changed. Steve had prostate cancer. The urologist explained that it was not all bad news. It was not all that much cancer, and the grade of the cancer was low. He recommended that Steve have surgery and said that he had an opening the following Wednesday.

Steve and Bonnie were stunned. How did this happen? They agreed to the surgery, Steve signed a pile of papers, and the next morning he went to see his boss to tell him that he needed time off.

His surgery took place the next Wednesday. He had never been admitted to a hospital before, and the three days he spent there were a blur of pain and nausea. It took him almost two days to realize that he had a catheter draining urine from his bladder, and he was shocked when he was told that he would go home with it in place. He hardly felt ready to go home, but he was discharged around lunchtime on Friday, and Bonnie drove him home. She had taken some time off work to look after him, and though he was grateful, he also felt like a little boy whose mommy had to take care of him.

Prostate cancer is typically a slow-growing cancer, so there is usually time for the man to think about the diagnosis and to plan for treatment. Steve was not given any treatment options, and he had very little preparation for the surgery. Surgery is just one of many options for localized prostate cancer. Other treatments include radiation (either external beam or brachytherapy), and for some men there is cryotherapy and experimental treatments such as HIFU (high intensity focused ultrasound). Although surgery has a good track record, it is certainly not the only treatment available.

Steve was home for six weeks. He was bored and irritable a lot of the time. He is just not someone who is used to sitting around. The catheter was removed ten days after the surgery, and this led to a major problem for him: he was leaking urine. At first he had no control, but over the next few weeks it got a bit better. After he came home, Bonnie bought him a pack of adult diapers, and he was very upset the first time he put one on. But it did the trick, and he was able to go for a walk. But he had to wear sweatpants, and he swore that everyone could see the big bulky diaper. By six weeks, he had some control, and he didn't wear the diapers anymore. He just went to the bathroom every hour or so, and that prevented major accidents. If he sneezed or coughed, he felt a gush of urine, and he spent a lot of time trying to figure out how he was going to go back to work with all of this happening.

Exactly six weeks after the surgery, he went back to see the urologist. The doctor looked at the incision on his stomach, nodded, and then told Steve he had "got it all." He also told him he could go back to work immediately. Steve seemed a bit shocked at this, but the doctor was in a hurry and ushered him out of the room. As Steve drove home, he tried to figure out how he was going to be able to work. He had to lift heavy beams and construction material, and there was not a toilet anywhere near where he was going to be working. Just thinking about it made his heart beat faster. But he had to do something; his leave from work was almost over.

Later that evening he talked to Bonnie about it. "What should I do, Bon? Can you imagine what it would be like, out on some job, and I have to go? And I'm up on the scaffolding? What will the guys say?"

"Oh, honey, I don't know. Maybe you can do something else on the site for a while. Have you talked to Jim? As the supervisor, he should know what you could do. There must be some other guy this has happened to."

"I guess I'll have to talk to him. I'll call him tomorrow. I just can't believe this has happened to me. It's such a mess."

Leakage of urine is a common problem after surgery for prostate cancer because the valve that keeps the bladder closed is destroyed when the prostate is removed. Different men experience the leakage in different ways. Some, like Steve, leak when they cough, sneeze, laugh, or make a sudden movement. Lifting something heavy can also cause leakage. Other men have constant dribbling. Some may try to empty their bladder regularly and at short intervals. This may prevent some leakage, but it is not the answer because a restroom is not always close by, and keeping the bladder empty does not solve the original problem.

The next day, Steve called Jim, the supervisor of the construction crew. He seemed happy to hear Steve's voice. "You coming back soon, big boy? The guys will be happy to see you! Me too. There's lots of work right now, and we need you, man."

"Um, that's good. It's just that . . . listen, can I come by the site and sit down and talk to you about something?"

"Sure, buddy. Anything serious? You sound kind of weird."

"Nah, I just want to talk to you in person. Can I come by tomorrow, maybe at the end of the day shift?"

"Sure. Say, 5:30 or so. See you, big boy!"

Steve smiled as he put the phone down. Jim was a great guy and easy to work with. He always had a smile on his face, and he made the guys feel important. Steve felt less nervous after hearing his voice, and he almost looked forward to going out to the work site to talk to him.

The next day went slowly for Steve. He wanted to go back to work and was eager to talk to Jim. But at the same time, he was afraid he wouldn't be able to do the work. He was also nervous about telling Jim about his leakage problem. What would he say? Would he tell the other guys? Steve knew he would be the laughing stock of the work site if anyone found out about his problem.

He left the house a bit early and got to the site with thirty minutes to spare before he was supposed to meet Jim. From the car he could see the building they were working on, and they had made a lot of progress in the six weeks he was at home. The building, an elementary school, was really taking shape. As he sat there, he saw his workmates finishing up for the day. Their mustard yellow coveralls were dirty, and most of them had taken off their hard hats, revealing their sweaty, messy hair. They came off the scaffolding and out of the building and walked toward the trailers where they would pick up their lunch kits and then head for their cars. Steve stayed in his car. He wasn't ready to face the rest of the guys just yet. When they had all driven off in their trucks and beat-up cars, Steve opened his car door and walked across the street to the trailer. The door was slightly open, and he could hear Jim talking on the phone. He pushed the door open, and Jim looked up and waved him over.

"Hey there, Steve! My man! How's it going?"

Jim stood up at his desk and reached out to shake Steve's hand. Jim's hand was rough and dry, and Steve suddenly felt ashamed that his hands had become soft in the time he had been away. "Hey, Jim. Good to see you. Looks like you've made good progress on the project. Are you on track for completion?"

"You bet! Things are a bit slower because my best guy was away, but if you're ready to come back, then we can get things going at full power again!"

Steve smiled, but then his face fell. He had to tell Jim the truth, and he just wasn't sure where to start. "So the doctor gave me the go-ahead to come back."

"Excellent!" Jim interrupted him. "Can I put you on the schedule for later this week?"

"Well, that's what I wanted to talk about. It's been tough being at home. Really boring, actually. And we could sure do with the money. It's just that . . ."

"Good, good!"

"It's just that I'm not sure I can do the work. I have this problem, you see, and it's really hard to talk about it, but . . ."

"Hey, say no more! I don't need the details. I really wanted you back, but if you can't do it, then you can't do it. I remember once working with another guy with cancer, and, well, let's just say it wasn't good. You don't have to work off any kind of notice or anything. Just get in touch with the HR folks at head office, and that'll be it. I'll be sorry to see you go, I can tell you, but if you can't work, you can't work."

Jim's tone was not friendly anymore. He barely made eye contact with Steve, and he seemed in a hurry to get rid of him. Steve opened his mouth to say something, but he could see that Jim had already moved on to something else. He was putting on his hard hat, and he had the walkie-talkie in his hand, ready to go out to the work site.

———∞———

There are over ten million cancer survivors in the United States today, and an estimated 3.8 million of them are adults who were employed at the time of their diagnosis and return to work after treatment. Some may even have worked throughout their treatment. Continuing to work is important for financial reasons, but also for self-esteem and social support. Returning to work is symbolic of having gotten through treatment and of a return to normality and stability. Many cancer survivors have to work to retain health insurance coverage, although their diagnosis may cause problems in that regard. On the other hand, a life-altering diagnosis can also prompt a reevaluation of priorities. Some people may choose to leave a job they do not enjoy to seek more satisfying employment, or they may take early retirement and focus on family and leisure activities instead of work.

Employers may assume that someone with cancer is no longer capable of carrying out their work as well as they did before. This may lead to discrimination, both subtle and overt, and cancer survivors have reported being dismissed, passed over for promotion, and denied benefits, as well as having experienced hostility in the workplace. All of these contravene the Americans with Disabilities Act, which was passed in 1990. People with cancer are included under this protection because cancer is regarded as a disease that impairs or limits a major life activity. The law, however, does not provide blanket coverage, and whether an employee is covered is decided on a case-by-case basis. Some courts have identified a weakness in the law: if a person with cancer is well enough to want to work, then they are not considered disabled.

———∞———

Steve followed Jim out of the trailer and walked quickly to his car. With each step he felt his anger rising until it spilled over just as he reached his car. He kicked the tire, and the pain in his foot brought him back to the problem. Jim had not even listened! He had just assumed that Steve couldn't work. He was not prepared to even hear him out. What was he going to do now? When he got home and walked in the door, Bonnie could see instantly that it had not gone well. She was preparing dinner, and she stopped as he slammed the kitchen door. She didn't say anything. She just stood there, a pile of sliced onions on the cutting board in front of her.

"Damn it, Bonnie! I'm not sure how much more of this I can take! First of all, I have to deal with the dribbling, and to cap it off, Jim thinks I'm not capable of working! He pretty much has me written off!"

"What did he say?"

"He told me that he'll miss me, but if I can't work, that's it. He didn't even listen! He just told me to get things sorted out with headquarters."

Bonnie had always been the more rational one, and she quickly thought of a solution. "Then deal with him at headquarters, Steve. They know the law. They'll do what's right by you. At the very least, they'll listen."

"So I'm expected to tell a complete stranger that I pee my pants?" Steve's voice was shaking with anger.

"No, honey, that's not what I said. Talk to the HR person, and tell them that you need some accommodation in your job. Maybe instead of doing all the lifting you could be doing more of the detail stuff. Remember I told you about that nurse who hurt her back? Well, she used to work on the labor floor, and they switched her to the clinic where she didn't have to do any heavy lifting."

"How is that the same as me?" Steve was getting angrier and angrier. He opened the refrigerator door, pulled out a beer, and slammed the door so hard the bottles on the shelves rattled loudly.

Bonnie knew that when he got like this, it was better to just leave him alone. She went back to slicing the onions, glad for an excuse for the tears that rolled down her cheeks. The past six weeks had been rough on her, too. She'd had to pick up extra shifts to make up for what he was not earning while he was on sick leave, and she was bone tired. She hated to see him so upset, but she was also a little irritated by his reaction. He often didn't stick up for himself at work, and then he whined to her afterward.

Dinner was quiet that evening. Neither of them seemed to want to start any conversation, so they ate in silence. Steve took his plate into the kitchen and then sat on the deck until it was dark. Bonnie left him to his thoughts, hoping he would sort things out in his head. She was asleep by the time he came up the stairs and into their bedroom. Neither of them slept well that night.

Steve was still asleep when Bonnie got up early the next morning. The Children's Hospital where she worked was a forty-five-minute drive from their house, and she hated the traffic, so she usually left just after six to avoid the snarls and slowdowns that were usual on the busy highway. Steve often worked the late shift, starting at noon, so he was usually asleep when Bonnie left. This morning was no different, except that Steve didn't have to go to work. Instead he got up at eight and called the HR department. He was a little surprised when someone answered the phone. The woman, Angela, told him that she was one of the counselors who could help him, and she suggested that he come in later that morning. Steve was not really prepared for this. He was hoping he could delay the meeting. But Angela insisted that she had time that morning, and she ended the call with a cheerful, "See you at eleven, then!"

Steve had not been to the new headquarters of the company. When he was hired, the company was just getting started, and they had a small run-down building on the outskirts of downtown. Now headquarters was located in a commercial park in the suburbs, and Steve whistled as he pulled into the parking lot. The building was big, really big. The entire structure was covered in blue black glass that shimmered in the morning sun. He could see rolling lawns at the back of the building flowing from a patio with tables and chairs, almost like a country club. The foyer was a light-filled expanse with an atrium that went up to skylights in the roof. In the middle was a huge reception desk with a very pretty young woman wearing headphones.

"Welcome to Bradley and Jones. How can I help you?"

"I'm here to see, um, someone in HR . . . something with an A."

"Angela Stone?"

Steve nodded, his face starting to color. What an idiot, he thought.

"One moment, please," and the young woman spoke softly into the mouthpiece that extended in front of her face.

"Ms. Stone will be down shortly. Please help yourself to an espresso while you wait." She pointed to a shiny machine that sat on a marble counter in the far corner of the atrium. It looked like a miniature Starbucks, with cups and plates and a big bowl of fruit. As he walked toward it, he heard his name called. He turned and saw another young woman walking in his direction with her hand outstretched.

"Steve? I'm Angela Stone, human resource counselor. We spoke earlier today. Nice to meet you."

Steve shook her hand, noticing that her grip was firm and her hand cool and dry.

"Can I help you with something to drink? That machine can be a bit tricky."

"Oh, no thank you. I was just checking it out. Fancy outfit, isn't it?"

"Sure is. Personally I think it's more for show than for use. Shall we go into one of our meeting rooms? It's just around this corner."

Steve felt himself start to whistle again. The building sure was something! In the old days, meetings were held anywhere there was space, sometimes out back standing around the flatbed of a truck. Now there were "meeting rooms" and fancy coffee machines.

Angela showed him into a small room with a round wooden table and two modern leather chairs. A fancy glass light fixture hung over the table, and a large mural covered one wall. The construction business must be good, he thought. They sat down in the leather chairs, and Angela pressed a button under the table. A computer screen rose out of a recess in the wooden tabletop. This time Steve whistled out loud. Angela smiled, punched in something on the hidden keyboard under the table, her eyes scanning whatever had appeared on the screen.

"So, Steve, you've been with Bradley and Jones for almost twenty years. Wow, you must be one of the originals! I see that you've been off on sick leave for six weeks and four days."

Steve had to force himself to keep his mouth closed.

"And where are you now? Are you ready to come back? No, wait, I see something here about a meeting you had with the site supervisor yesterday."

Steve had to jump in. "Yes, I met with Jim. I had this surgery, you see, cancer surgery, and I'm not sure that I can do the same kinds of things I did before. So I went to talk to him, and he told me I was finished with the company. Just like that, after twenty years!"

"Hang on a minute, Steve. I'm not sure what happened at that meeting, but it sure sounds like you think you're fired. Jim can't fire you. Only I can fire you!" She saw the look on his face. "I was just trying to make a joke. Not even I can fire you, and there is no plan to fire you. Tell me about what's going on with you, and let's see what we can do."

Steve drew in a deep breath. Something in his gut told him that this woman could help him, and he decided he was going to lay it on the line for her. He was going to trust her and hope it paid off.

"Okay, so I was diagnosed with prostate cancer about two months ago, and I had the surgery. The doc says they got it all, and I'm fine. Well, the cancer part is fine. It's just that I have this problem." His voice faltered for a second, but the look on her face was one of kindness and sympathy, so he started again.

"Anyway, since the surgery, I have this problem with . . . well, it's a problem with using the restroom. Oh, this is so weird, talking to a stranger about this. But anyway, if I'm not close to a restroom, I can have an accident. Not like an accident with the building, but an accident, you know, down there." He could no longer look at Angela, and his shoulders slumped as he looked at his feet.

"So you're having some problems with your bladder?" she asked softly.

His head shot up and he looked at her with wide eyes. "How did you know?"

"My dad is a prostate cancer survivor. Ten years now. And I remember what he went through. He was older than you, I think, in his late fifties, but it sure bothered him. He went through a bit of a depression to tell you the truth. But it got better, and now he's back to his old self, maybe even better. So let's talk about what you will need in order to make it possible for you to work."

Steve was stunned. She knew! She understood! They talked for a while about how the company could accommodate him. She asked a lot of questions, and as they talked, he found it easier and easier to answer her questions. She explained a lot, too, about the law and what companies had to reasonably do to ensure that employees could go back to their old jobs, or to find something that they could do in a new position. For the first time in many weeks, Steve felt better, really better.

———

Under the Americans with Disabilities Act (ADA), an employer with more than fifteen employees must make reasonable accommodation for workers with a disability, as long as this does not impose an "undue hardship" on the company's business. Undue hardship is defined as anything that requires significant difficulty or expense in light of the company's size or resources. The employer is also not required to lower quality or production standards in making the accommodation or to provide personal-use items such as hearing aids for an employee.

The ADA prohibits discrimination in hiring or firing employees and in the provision of benefits. Reasonable accommodations that should be made for employees with cancer include changes in work hours or time off for medical appointments and side effects from treatment. Most accommodations for workers do not cost money, and if they do, the amount is usually very little, around $500.

The Family and Medical Leave Act (FMLA) pertains to companies with over fifty employees. Under this act, the company must allow twelve weeks of unpaid leave during any twelve-month period, and it requires the company to continue to provide benefits, including health insurance, during the leave period. The employee must be allowed to return to the same or an equivalent position after the leave. FMLA also allows leave to care for a spouse, child, or parent with a serious health condition and for a reduced work schedule when medically necessary.

———

Steve felt about twenty pounds lighter after talking with Angela, and the weight came off his shoulders and head. He could even breathe better. During their discussion, Steve realized that what he needed to be able to work was easy access to a restroom and, for the next while, a slightly altered workload with limited lifting. They talked about whether he was comfortable staying on the same job and reporting to Jim. This caused Steve to hesitate for a moment. Would Jim accept him? And what about the other guys? Angela sensed his uncertainty about this.

"What's the worst thing that could happen if you go back to that job?"

"Well, I guess Jim could make it really unpleasant for me. I could end up with all the shit—oh, excuse my language—jobs, and then he would really have an excuse to fire me if I couldn't do them."

"Remember that he can't fire you, Steve," Angela prompted him. "But okay, let's say he gives you jobs to do that you aren't comfortable doing. What then?"

"Well, I guess I could call you in."

"Yes, you could. I think what we should do is have a meeting with Jim. Explain to him what the plan is, and allow him to express any concerns he has. And then you could both talk to the guys on the site. From our end, we'll get a portable restroom installed close to the building so you don't have to walk too far to relieve yourself. I'll set up the meeting with Jim for this week, and I'll call you with the date and time. How about you plan on being back at work after we meet with Jim and discuss your needs? Does that sound okay?"

Steve drove home with the windows down and the radio blaring his favorite hard rock station. He could hardly wait for Bonnie to come home so he could tell her the good news. When he got home, he felt so good that he tidied the kitchen, mopped the floors, and started dinner. Bonnie was going to be surprised! And she was. She noticed how clean the kitchen was the moment she came in the door. It smelled of a combination of lemons from the soap he had used to clean the floor and garlic from the pot simmering on the stove. Steve also looked happier than he had in ages.

"What happened?" she asked, her smile making her words sound hopeful.

"I saw this great woman named Angela at headquarters. She was amazing, really supportive and helpful. We're going to talk to Jim, and I'm going back to work!"

"That's great, honey! I'm really happy she could help. When did you see her? When do you think you'll be back at work?"

"I saw her this morning. She was really nice. She said I could go back to work after we've talked to Jim. She's going to set up a meeting with me and Jim so we can talk about what I can do and what I can't do. She's also going to get one of those portable potty things so it'll be closer to where I'm working."

Bonnie had to smile again. When she had suggested that he tell his employer about his problem with his bladder, he had blown up at her. Now it was all fine, and this Angela person had saved the day. Part of her wanted to say "I told you so," but that was really not the point. He was happier than he had been in a really long time, and that made her happy. They opened a bottle of wine with dinner that night, and afterward they sat out on the deck, watching the sky change colors from blue to black.

The next morning, Steve called Angela. He had to leave a voice message because her line was busy, but almost immediately after he put the phone down, she called him back.

"How about you meet me at the job site this afternoon? I talked to Jim, and we're going to meet at four o'clock. Are you free?"

"I am nothing but free!" he laughed. "Thanks for all your help, Angela. You've been amazing!"

Steve paced the house for most of the day until he left for the job site. His heart was beating fast, but it was with excitement this time. He pulled into the parking lot next to the school they were building. From the car, he could hear the whining of saws and the clanging of hammers against steel. It sounded like music to his ears, and he realized again how much he missed work. He looked around to see if Angela had arrived yet. The parking lot was full of trucks and dirty cars, all of them he recognized as belonging to his workmates. And then in the rearview mirror he saw a shiny new car entering the parking lot. That had to be Angela, so he got out of his car to greet her. She was wearing high heels, and she took her time negotiating the gravel lot with its uneven surface. She looked a little embarrassed that he was watching her, and she was laughing when she eventually reached him.

"I should have thought a bit more about my fashion statement this morning! Good afternoon, Steve. Are you ready?"

Steve nodded. "More than I've ever been."

She knocked loudly on the door of the trailer and pushed the door open. Jim was sitting at his desk, his boots resting just to the side of the computer keyboard. He was talking on the phone, and he quickly leaped to his feet when he saw Angela. He put down the phone in a hurry, wiped his hands on his overalls, and nodded to Steve in greeting.

"Jim, you know Steve, right?" began Angela. "As you know, I'm Angela Stone from company headquarters. I'm here today to facilitate a meeting with you two to discuss Steve's return to work at this site. I know that you two met earlier this week, and there seems to have been some misunderstanding. But that's bygones. Today we're going to talk about what we need to do as a company to make sure that Steve here can continue to be a part of the team. Okay?"

Jim seemed a bit taken aback. He nodded and sat down, ignoring the fact that there was only one chair in front of his desk. Steve quickly turned around and looked for another chair. There wasn't one. He did see a large plastic pail in the corner, so he dragged that over and sat on it while Angela took the only chair. It was dusty, but she didn't seem to notice or mind.

"So, Jim, let's begin. Steve is anxious to get back to work, and he has the all clear from his doctor. From my discussion with him, there seem to be two areas where we, you, have to modify things a bit. Steve should ease back into heavy lifting, so for the next while, he should not be doing any of that. Can you make that work?"

Jim hesitated, trying to figure out in his head what that would mean for the job.

"How have you been managing with him not here for the past six weeks? Did you hire a replacement worker?"

"Well, no. The other guys just picked up the slack. But they're not going to be happy if he comes back and there's not much he can do."

Steve bristled. This was just what he was afraid of. "But there's plenty I can do. You've made a lot of progress. You told me you were on target. There's tons of other stuff to be done now, stuff that I can do easily!"

"Well, yes, but what will the guys say when you get special treatment?" Jim countered, his face getting red with irritation.

"Hang on a moment, guys!" Angela interrupted. "There are rules about this. Jim, it's your job to make sure the rest of the crew understands that Steve won't be doing any heavy lifting. You also have to make sure that there's work for him that he *can* do. This is not a matter of choice. The law says you have to do this!"

Jim glared at her. Steve felt a twinge in his stomach. This was not going well. And she still had to tell him about the portable toilet.

"How about you set up a meeting with the rest of the crew, and I'll be there to back you up when you tell them about Steve coming back to work? You can make it seem like this is coming from up above, orders from headquarters. That might make it better."

Jim thought about this for a moment and then nodded his head. "We usually have a quick meeting first thing on Monday mornings to talk about the work plan for the week. It's early, though, seven o'clock at the start of the first shift. You think you can make it that early?"

Angela laughed at the supervisor, but in a kind way. "Is that a challenge? You think this little lady can't get up that early? I'm at the gym by six most mornings, so you don't scare me!"

They all laughed, and the tension in the trailer lessened a bit. Steve was still nervous about the toilet, but he wasn't going to bring up the topic and Angela hadn't said anything.

"Okay, so I'll be here bright and early on Monday morning. Seven, did you say? Now, how about you show me around the site? I bet Steve would like to see how the job's going."

"Sure thing. You're going to need a hard hat, and those shoes aren't exactly safe."

"Give me the hat, and don't worry about the shoes. I can run a mile in these things."

There are different ways of planning your return to work. The kind of work you do plays a role, as does how well your recovery from treatment is progressing. We know that people who do physical work, particularly if there is heavy lifting involved, often have a more difficult time returning to work.

It is important to start making plans before your sick leave is over. Although it is important to get the "all clear" from your treating physician, it is also important to consult someone who understands the issues related to the work you do. An occupational health specialist can be very helpful in this regard. Your company or insurance plan may have someone you can speak to before you go back to work. The specialist will usually assess your physical and emotional health and ask questions about the kind of work you do, the work environment, and other factors that may impact your return to work.

It is helpful to have a plan in writing that you draw up with your supervisor and the occupational health specialist. The plan needs to clearly describe how many hours you can work, the kind of work you will be doing, how your work hours will increase over time if you are on a graduated back-to-work program, and the proposed date when you will be back at work or working full time.

Evaluate this plan with your supervisor every two weeks and adjust as needed. You may be able to speed up the plan, or you may have to alter it to allow more time on a reduced workload. If the plan is not working for you or your supervisor, you may have to draw up a revised work plan that is more realistic.

It is also important to let your coworkers know that you are on a back-to-work plan so that they will understand that you are not slacking off but rather are working reduced hours for a certain period of time or have made adjustments to your role. Transparency can prevent a lot of problems.

The three of them stepped out of the trailer and onto the path that led to the school building. The concrete walls were up, and most of the scaffolding had been removed. Steve knew from experience that the roof would go up next, and he felt the usual excitement at that stage of the process. Most of the guys were working inside the building now, and the trio entered the building cautiously, careful not to step in any puddles or gaps in the floor. A couple of the guys waved to Steve when they saw him, stopping for a few moments from their welding or drilling to raise a free hand in greeting. Steve inhaled the smells of concrete and steel and felt at home. Angela asked a lot of questions, mostly of Jim, and the supervisor bent his head to talk into her ear. The construction site was a symphony of loud noises, and Angela strained to hear his answers.

After about twenty minutes, the tour was complete. Steve was amazed at how much they had done in the time he had been away. His long experience in the construction world allowed him to see where he could pitch in. There was still lots to do. As they walked back to the trailer, their hard hats in their hands, Angela continued to ask questions.

"Jim, tell me something. This may seem like a weird question, but where do the guys go to relieve themselves? The restrooms for the school aren't ready yet, and somehow I can't see these big guys using those itty-bitty toilets for the kids."

Blushing, Jim laughed and then answered. "Well, they usually just go on their breaks. There's a coffee shop about half a block from here in one direction and a gas station about a block the other way."

"Really?" Angela's tone was surprised. "You have nothing on site? That seems a bit harsh to me, even for a bunch of tough construction guys! In the summer you guys must drink a lot, too, to keep hydrated. That must make things difficult."

Steve had to hide his smile. She sure was smart! He could see where she was going with this, and a wave of gratitude flowed through him. She was going to solve his problem and not let Jim or the guys know it was his problem!

"Well, it's always been that way on the job," explained Jim. "I've never had a complaint, either. That's just the way it's been."

"Well, I'm sure we can do something about that to make it better for all of you. I'm going to order a portable toilet that they'll set up close to the building. We're probably breaking all sorts of labor laws with the present situation, so please don't say a word!"

She laughed, and Jim let out a short chuckle. She handed her hard hat back to him, shook his free hand, and started walking back to her car. Steve watched her go, her high heels sinking slightly into the gravel with each step. But she kept on going, and she waved at them when she reached her car. Steve left Jim and went inside the trailer to put his hard hat away. Monday was only four days away, and he felt excited at the prospect of being back at work. It was just a few days.

Why Do I Feel So Tired?

*M*any survivors assume that once treatment is over they will feel "normal" again. They may be surprised when side effects linger for a long time. In this chapter, you will meet Barb who is surprised that six months after treatment for uterine cancer she is still tired and sore.

Barbara had recently retired as a teacher after almost thirty-five years at the same school. She was known as Miss B. to most of the people in town. She loved her job and the two generations of children that had come and gone in her classroom. Living in a small town outside Chicago, she knew the parents and grandparents of most of her students. She loved seeing the children grow up, even though when they were in high school they looked embarrassed to see her. They would mostly disappear for their college years, and then many of them would come back to raise families of their own. Barbara had never married or had children of her own, so her students, past and present, were the closest thing to family for her.

She lived in a small house about two blocks from the school and took great pride in her garden. Beginning in the spring, she would spend the late afternoons there, digging weeds and later deadheading the flowers. Her roses had won the blue ribbon in the state fair in 1999. At fifty-nine years of age, she was content with her life. She had friends in town as well as in Chicago, and because she had been careful with her money over the years, she was able to take a cruise every winter. Life was good. Like all of her friends, she had gone through menopause in the past ten years. She'd had it easier than some of them who complained incessantly about hot flashes and weight gain. Barbara felt that they enjoyed moaning about it. She was of the opinion that this was a natural part of life and that one should just get on with things and ignore the small stuff. She was very surprised one afternoon

63

in the early winter to discover that she was bleeding. There was a big stain in her underwear. What was this all about? She had not had a period for almost ten years, so this was very surprising. She was busy packing for her annual cruise, and for a moment she almost panicked. But then, being the sensible person she was, she shook her head, took a deep breath, and went back to what she was doing. It was nothing; she was sure of it. She was leaving the next day for Chicago, where she would spend the night with her friend Joan, and the following day the two of them were flying to the coast to board the ship. She kept checking in the bathroom, and the bleeding seemed to have stopped. So she went to bed, excited about the cruise.

She arrived in Chicago just after lunch the following day, and she and Joan had a lovely evening together. They went to a small restaurant near Joan's apartment, and they each had two glasses of wine, enough to make them tipsy and giggly. What fun they were going to have on the cruise! It was a new ship, too, and they had already planned out most of their activities for the ten-day voyage around the Caribbean. There were bridge classes and big musical productions, and Joan was planning to do the early morning yoga class every day. Their flight to Fort Lauderdale was uneventful, and early in the afternoon they boarded the big white ship.

The ten days flew by really fast. The ship was everything they had read about in the glossy brochures. It was beautiful, with luxurious state rooms and multiple restaurants, and you could be busy twenty-four hours a day with activities. Barbara and Joan had traveled together before, and they got along really well. Joan was more outgoing than Barbara, and she made her friend do things she would not normally do. Barbara quite enjoyed this. With Joan around, she could be someone other than the quiet retired teacher.

The only thing that marred an otherwise perfect cruise was the spotting that Barbara continued to experience on the ship. She even had to go to the ship's pharmacy to buy some panty liners. She was now getting worried, and one afternoon she went to the ship's Internet café and logged on to search for information. What she read scared her. All of the websites suggested that any bleeding after menopause was suspicious and needed to be investigated. She almost made an appointment right then and there to see the ship's physician, but she knew that was just silly. She needed to see her own health care provider, and she planned to do that just as soon as she got home. She thought about calling the clinic from the ship to make an appointment for the day she returned home but decided it was too expensive. So she waited and worried. The last two days of the cruise were wasted on her. All she could think about was what was wrong with her, and she checked her underwear every hour. Joan looked at her with what looked like suspicion every time she excused herself to go to the restroom, but they were both too polite to ask or explain anything.

They had a three-hour wait at the Fort Lauderdale airport before catching their flight back to Chicago. While they were sitting and waiting for their flight, Joan asked Barbara what was wrong.

"Something's going on with you, Barbara. Are you okay?"

Barbara's face went red, and she felt the tears rush into her eyes. "Oh, Joan. I'm so worried. All the time we were on the cruise I've had this . . . oh, this is so embarrassing! I've been bleeding, you know, down there. I looked it up on the Internet, and I'm scared it's something bad."

"Oh dear. What are you going to do?"

"Well, I'm going to see my nurse practitioner as soon as I can. What else can I do? I'm scared, Joan, really scared. I've tried to be healthy all my life, and now this. How could this happen to me?"

Joan looked at her friend. She didn't look like someone who'd been on a relaxing cruise. Her face was pinched and her shoulders were tense.

"Well, don't panic until you know for sure. Do you want me to see if my gynecologist will see you? How much do you trust this nurse of yours?"

"I trust Jenny completely! She's a lovely young woman, married to one of my students. She'll get to the bottom of this, I'm sure. She takes really good care of me. She always reminds me to have my mammogram, and she spends as much time as I need every time I see her. She'll know what to do!"

As she defended herself and her nurse practitioner, Barbara realized that she had faith in her health care provider and that perhaps she was getting all worked up without any evidence that something bad was happening to her. She felt herself relax just a little bit, and she even managed to doze on the flight to Chicago. They arrived in the middle of the afternoon, and Barbara decided not to spend the night at Joan's apartment as they had originally planned but rather to catch the first train back home. The hour-long train ride seemed like it took a day, and it was dark when she finally unlocked the front door of her little house.

It was too late to call the clinic, and Barbara spent the rest of the evening unpacking and doing laundry. She slept poorly and was awake at 5 a.m. Then she paced her house until it was time to call the clinic. Something in her voice must have alerted the receptionist, who gave her an appointment for just after lunch the same day. That was four hours away, and Barbara found herself watching the clock in the kitchen as the hands slowly circled the numbers. She thought about going to the store to pick up milk and bread, but she couldn't face anyone asking about her vacation. So she ate some dry cereal right out of the box and waited for the minutes and hours to tick by.

She was startled when she heard a key in the front door, and then she remembered that she was only due home that day, and it was probably her neighbor coming to check on things as they had arranged. It was indeed her neighbor, a young woman named Sue who lived next door with her boyfriend. Sue was carrying a brown paper bag from the grocery store, and she nearly dropped it when she saw Barbara in the kitchen.

"Oh my goodness, you scared me!" she burst out. "What are you doing here?"

"I came home last night. Sorry, I should have called you, but I forgot. Thank you so much for looking after the house while I was away. Everything is just perfect."

"It's my pleasure. I went to the store and bought you some basics, just some milk and juice, and they had some nice ripe bananas."

"Thank you so much, Sue. How much do I owe you? That was very thoughtful of you."

"Oh, please don't worry about paying me back. It's my pleasure. Think of it as payback for all the green beans and tomatoes you gave us last summer! I can't stop now—I have to go and change my clothes. I have a job interview this morning, for a teacher's assistant position at the school. Wouldn't it be amazing if I got the job? I could come and ask you for advice! Wish me luck!"

And with that she left Barbara sitting in the kitchen, deep in thought. It was almost eleven o'clock. She had almost two hours to fill before she could leave for the clinic, which was just three blocks away. It was cold, but she thought she would walk there. The fresh air would do her good, and it would give her time to think about what she was going to say to the nurse practitioner. The bleeding had almost stopped now, with just the occasional stain on her panty liner, but she knew that something was wrong, and she wanted to find out what was happening to her.

She ate one of the bananas that Sue had brought her for lunch and set off down the road a full thirty minutes before her appointment. She hated all this waiting! From a block away, she could see that the parking lot of the clinic was empty—it was lunchtime, and the clinic was closed for an hour—and she hoped someone would let her in and not leave her out on the step in the cold. The front door of the clinic was indeed open, and there was a sign on the reception desk that said the staff was on their break and to please take a seat. She did as instructed, sitting in one of the armchairs in the corner of the waiting room. There was a houseplant on the side table next to her chair, and she stared at it as she waited. It was a pathetic specimen, starving for sunlight and water. She couldn't stop herself from cleaning the poor thing up. First she picked off all the leaves that were dry and curled up at the edges. There was a plastic card holder stuck in the dried-out dirt in the pot, and she used that to stab around the roots and loosen the dirt. She was about to take the whole thing to the restroom to give it some water when she heard the receptionist return to her desk.

"Barbara? Barbara Mason?"

Barbara looked up from what she was doing. Before she could reply, the receptionist motioned for her to come around the side of the desk. Barbara put down the plant, walked to where the receptionist was waiting for her, and followed her down the long hallway. She was familiar with the layout of the clinic and knew that Jenny the nurse practitioner used the very last examination room. She sat down in the chair next to the desk and waited for Jenny to arrive. She could hear her hurried footsteps coming down the hallway. Jenny was always in a rush, and yet she managed to make her patients feel like she had all the time in the world for them.

The door of the examination room opened, and Jenny entered the room. She was in her early thirties, with curly red hair and a face full of freckles. She always seemed to be in a good mood, and today was no different. Her smile was wide and bright as she greeted Barbara.

"Hi there, Barbara! How are you? Just back from your vacation, I gather. Did you get sick on the ship?"

Barbara did not know where to begin. She wished it was something as simple as a stomach bug or a cold. But then she wouldn't have come to see Jenny.

"I don't really know how to begin. It's very embarrassing, really."

"Just take your time. I've heard all sorts of things, and the patient is always more embarrassed than me."

"Well, just before I went away, I had some bleeding, you know, down there."

"Okay. So you had some vaginal bleeding. You went through menopause some time ago, right? So tell me more about this. How much bleeding? How long did it last?"

Jenny's matter-of-fact attitude helped Barbara to relax, and she soon found herself describing exactly what had happened over the past two weeks.

"I'm going to need to examine you, Barbara, and depending on what I can see or feel, we'll make some plans. I'd like you to undress from the waist down and lie on the exam table. I'll be back in a few minutes."

Barbara did as she was asked and lay on the hard examination table until Jenny came back. The draw sheet covering her legs felt cool, and she could sense the goose bumps along her bare shins. Jenny knocked on the door before entering. Barbara had an internal exam every year, but she still felt apprehensive. Jenny was gentle in both her manner and her touch, and it was over in just a few minutes. Once again, Jenny left the room while her patient got back into her clothes. When she returned, her smile was not as wide.

"I couldn't feel anything on examination, Barbara, but any bleeding after menopause is not normal. I am going to refer you to a gynecologist for an endometrial biopsy. What this involves is taking a specimen of tissue from the lining of your uterus. The procedure itself is quite quick, but you may have some bleeding afterward. I can send you to Dr. Smithers here in town or to a larger clinic in Chicago. Do you have a preference?"

Barbara did not hesitate. Bill Smithers was a childhood friend of her brother's. He used to tease her about anything and everything, and there was no way she was going to allow him to do anything to her. She knew it was silly. They were both much older now, and he was a professional, but she just could not imagine him touching her.

"I think I'd like to go to Chicago, Jenny. I was doing some reading on the Internet, and if this is cancer, and I think we both know there's a good chance it is, I'd prefer to be treated in the city. Is that okay?"

"Of course! Don't you worry about a thing. I'll send in that referral this afternoon, and hopefully you'll be seen early next week. You'll probably want to stay overnight in Chicago. Do you have friends or relatives in the city?"

Barbara assured Jenny that she could stay with any one of her friends. She went home with no real answer to her fears, but with a plan that she knew would lead to answers. Two days later, she received a call from a gynecologist's office in downtown Chicago. They had an opening for the following Monday afternoon. Barbara called Joan and asked if she could stay over that night. Now she just had to get through the weekend.

As the nurse practitioner explained to Barbara, any vaginal bleeding after menopause needs to be investigated. A transvaginal ultrasound is a test where the inside of the uterus is examined to see if the lining is thickened. Women who have gone through menopause should have a thin lining in the uterus. Additional information can be gathered from taking a small piece of the uterine lining and examining it under a high-powered microscope to look for evidence of cancer.

The weekend passed slowly, and on Monday morning Barbara took the train into Chicago. It was a very different journey than the one she had taken before the start of her cruise. She was worried, very worried, and a bit afraid of what the procedure would be like. She had never gone to a doctor in the big city, and she felt intimidated. Would they treat her like a country bumpkin? Jenny and the other medical staff at the clinic in her town were always so nice. She was not sure that these city people would be the same way. She found the gynecologist's office quite easily. It was on a side street that linked busy

Michigan Avenue with Lakeshore Drive. She had probably walked down this same street before on one of her visits to the city, but this time her heart was beating fast with fear as she walked toward the shiny glass doors. She had to take the elevator to the fifteenth floor, and her stomach was queasy as the elevator ascended with a whoosh. The office was very fancy, and this didn't help to put her at ease. But the receptionist was friendly, and she didn't have to wait at all. She was ushered into an examination room that had all kinds of equipment in it. She undressed and put on a gown made of soft pink cotton, so different from the paper ones at her usual clinic.

There was a knock on the door just as she finished folding her clothes neatly. A young woman dressed in scrubs entered the room.

"Hello. I'm Dr. Moody, the gynecologist you've been referred to. I hope you haven't been waiting long. I know how irritating that can be. So, Ms. Mason, tell me a little bit about your symptoms."

Barbara went through the whole story again. She was getting a bit irritated with having to repeat things over and over. Why didn't they just send proper notes to each other? The doctor asked more questions, and then it was time for the biopsy. Barbara could feel herself tensing up in anticipation of the pain as she lay down on the examination table and put her feet into the cold footrests at the end of the table. The doctor had to tell her three times to relax and open her knees. Barbara was really trying, but she was scared and felt out of control of her own body.

Dr. Moody explained what she was doing as she was doing it. This helped Barbara a bit, and within just a few minutes, with what felt like two pinches, it was over. The doctor started telling Barbara what would happen next, but she was not really listening. Her head was whirling with all sorts of thoughts, and the doctor's voice was merely a droning sound in the background. Barbara couldn't wait to get out of there. She struggled to sit up, and in the process the sheet of paper that had been over her knees fell to the floor. She was left on the examination table half naked and embarrassed beyond belief. On her way out of the office, her face still flushed and her eyes not making contact with anyone, someone handed her a small card with the date and time for the follow-up appointment. Barbara put it in her pocket and left the office as quickly as she could.

She found the card with the appointment two days later when she was putting on her coat and its sharp edges pressed against her fingers. The appointment was just three days away! Once again she traveled by train to the city, walked down the street to the doctor's office, and went up the elevator to the fifteenth floor. This time she was ushered into the gynecologist's office, and she sat in a plush chair before a modern steel and glass desk, waiting to hear her fate. The gynecologist walked into the office with a file in her hand.

When she looked up and greeted Barbara, Barbara could see from the expression on her face that it was bad.

"Ms. Mason. Not good news, I'm afraid. The biopsy showed endometrial cancer—uterine cancer—and you're going to need surgery. This is a very curable cancer, I assure you, but it's cancer nonetheless."

Barbara felt herself go cold, an icy cold that started inside her chest and spread outward to her hands and feet and head. "When? Where? How soon can you do this?"

"I'll have to check my schedule, but I do surgery every Tuesday and Thursday. So I could operate probably within the next couple of weeks. I see that you live outside of Chicago. Do you have friends or family here in the city with whom you could spend a couple of days recuperating?"

Barbara nodded, her head spinning as she tried to think about everything she had to do and how she was going to manage.

Endometrial cancer is a common cancer in women, affecting the lining of the uterus. It is usually diagnosed at an early stage because the early warning signs are quite obvious. Any bleeding from the uterus after menopause is regarded as suspicious.

This cancer is usually treated with surgical removal of the whole uterus, an operation called a hysterectomy. The uterine tubes and ovaries are usually removed during the surgery, as well, and lymph nodes in the area are checked and samples are sent for examination. Surgical removal of the uterus is usually curative. However, some women do need radiation therapy, hormone therapy, or chemotherapy if there is a risk that the cancer has spread to other parts of the body or is an aggressive form that may spread in the future.

The days flew by. Barbara spent most of the time in Chicago. She had different appointments in preparation for the surgery, and it was just easier to stay with Joan in the city. The following Thursday morning she was admitted to the hospital where she had the surgery. She stayed in the hospital for about three days, most of it a fog of pain and delicious release when she was given pain medication. The day she was discharged, as she waited for Joan to escort her back to her apartment, Dr. Moody came to say good-bye.

"I have the preliminary pathology results back, Barbara. I think I'm going to send you to a cancer specialist for an expert opinion. There were aspects of the tumor that look more aggressive to the pathologist, and I think some radiation treatment would be a good idea. But we'll sort that all out when you come back to see me in about four weeks, okay? Just go home and get some rest. We'll deal with all of this when you are fully recovered."

More bad news! When Joan arrived, she found Barbara sitting on the bed, her shoulders slumped and a soggy Kleenex in her hand. Her eyes were red from crying, and she sniffed every few seconds. Joan put her arms around her friend and gave her a long hug.

"Whatever it is, you'll get through it. You'll see. You're a strong woman, and you've got friends who love you. It'll be okay. It'll be okay."

"I have to have more treatment! The doctor was just here, and I have to have radiation too! Why did this have to happen to me? Why?"

She started to sob in earnest, her shoulders moving up and down in the arms of her friend. And now she was embarrassed to be acting like a big baby in front of Joan. After a few minutes, she stopped crying, blew her nose with a loud honk, and stood up.

"I have to get out of here, Joan. Please take me home—to your place, I mean. I just have to get out of this hospital and away from all of this!"

They went to Joan's apartment, slowly because Barbara still had pain from the incision on her abdomen. She held on to Joan's arm as they negotiated the hallways of the hospital and went out to a taxi. She spent the next week at Joan's, resting and sleeping and reading when she had the energy. Ten days after her surgery, she was feeling well enough to go back to her own home. Joan was worried about her and wanted her to stay longer, but Barbara needed desperately to be back at home. So she took the train, and her steps were slow and measured as she walked back up the path to her beloved little house.

Her neighbor Sue had once again taken excellent care of everything. A pile of mail—cards wishing her well from many of her friends and acquaintances in the town—waited for her on the hall stand. There was fresh milk and bread in the kitchen and a lovely bouquet of flowers on the table. Barbara stayed home for the next three weeks. She had many visitors and a fridge and freezer full of meals that people brought over. She hadn't realized how much support she had in the town, even after all the years she had lived there and all the people she had come in contact with as a teacher. She was almost happy except for the twinges of fear she felt every now and then as she anticipated what would come next. She had an appointment with Dr. Moody exactly five weeks later, and someone had called from a Dr. Bloom's office with an appointment for the same afternoon. She thought this must be the cancer specialist, and she asked Joan to go with her to both of these appointments. She needed the company and support.

Her appointment with Dr. Moody was brief. The doctor looked at her incision, which had healed well. She then told Barbara that the pathology had confirmed the fact that it was an aggressive kind of cancer and that she was going to need radiation therapy.

"I have an appointment this afternoon with Dr. Bloom. Is he the radiation specialist?"

"Yes, Dr. Bloom is a radiation oncologist. But she's a woman, one of my classmates from medical school. She's very nice, and she works at a wonderful cancer center. You'll get very good care there."

Joan had been holding her hand as they sat in Dr. Moody's office. She didn't let go as they left the building and climbed into a cab that took them to the cancer center in another part of the city. Barbara could feel her heart fluttering in her chest, and she was sure that if Joan had not been holding her hand, she would have taken off out of the seat. She knew she was being silly, but she was very afraid. She was still tired after the surgery even though she had hardly done anything for herself for the past five weeks. Everyone had taken such good care of her, but she was not sleeping well and she had little appetite.

The cab arrived outside a large building covered in blue glass. Barbara drew in a deep breath as she and Joan got out of the cab. This was it.

"Just hang onto my hand and squeeze if you feel overwhelmed." Joan had thankfully taken charge. "Now, let's find out where this Dr. Bloom is."

There was a large reception desk just inside the glass doors, and a friendly young woman directed them to the elevators and down into the basement.

"Oh, that doesn't sound good," mumbled Barbara. "Why the basement?"

"Probably because they usually have the radiation machines in the basement where they have very thick walls." Joan had worked in a doctor's office before she retired, and she knew a lot about all sorts of medical things.

Once again they had to check in at a reception desk. This time they were shown to some chairs in a crowded waiting room where they waited and waited. Barbara could feel her anxiety rising as the minutes ticked by. There was a large clock on the wall, and she watched the second hand inch its way around the face, over and over again. Eventually she heard her name called. It was almost forty minutes past her appointment time, and she was now more annoyed than anxious. Joan hesitated for a moment when Barbara stood up, but Barbara reached down and took her friend's hand.

"You're coming with me, to stop me from yelling more than anything else. How can they be so inefficient?"

The two women followed a young man who was dressed in a loose cotton top and pants. He had introduced himself, but Barbara was distracted by her irritation and hadn't listened. He showed them into a small examination room, and Joan looked around.

"I really do think I should leave, Barb. There's not much room in here."

"Don't you leave me! Stay!"

Their conversation was interrupted by the hurried entrance of a young woman in a white coat. She was out of breath, her curly hair escaping from a loose bun at the back of her neck.

"I'm so sorry to have kept you waiting, Mrs., um, Ms. Moody. I'm Dr. Bloom. I got a late start this morning. The babysitter didn't show up, and I've been playing catch-up ever since. But that's not any of your concern. You're here to see me, and for the next little while you'll have my full attention. Let's get started, shall we?"

She barely glanced at Joan who was standing next to Barbara because there was only one chair in the room. As she sat down on a stool with wheels, she read from a piece of paper that was stapled to the cardboard chart in her hands.

"Ah, right. This is a referral from Melinda Moody. Pretty straightforward, really. We're going to give you some radiation to the pelvis to make sure all the cancer is gone. You'll have daily treatments, not on the weekends of course, and you should be done in about four weeks or so. Before we start, you'll meet with my assistant, and she'll fill you in on all the details. It's been a pleasure to meet you. Any questions?"

Barbara felt like she had been hit over the head. Of course she had questions! But she didn't know what they were yet. Even Joan seemed stunned and just stood there with a puzzled expression on her face. Dr. Bloom smiled pleasantly and exited the room, leaving the two women in silence. Within just a few minutes, there was a soft knock at the door. An older woman entered the room. She wore a brightly colored cotton jacket over pale pink scrubs.

"Hello, I'm Irene, one of the nurses here. Which one of you is Ms. Mason?"

"You can't tell?" burst out Joan, her exasperation clearly showing. "This is Ms. Mason, the one who looks like she was just hit over the head!"

"Sorry about Dr. Bloom. She's been running late all morning, and she gets a bit flustered. I'm here to give you some information about what will happen next. I have some reading material for you, too, but why don't we just sit and chat for a while?"

And Irene sat with them for the next forty-five minutes, patiently explaining what would happen over the course of Barbara's treatment. She answered their questions and even drew some diagrams to help them understand. Her calm demeanor really helped, and she even managed to make Barbara laugh once or twice. Both women felt much more confident when they finally finished, and Barbara knew that she could call Irene when she needed more information during her treatment. As Irene escorted them out of the examination room, she introduced them to a young man passing in the hallway. His name was Tom, and he was one of the radiation therapists who would actually be doing the treatment. He greeted them warmly and told Barbara that he was looking forward to getting to know her better over the next few weeks. What a difference from the hurried doctor!

Preparing for treatment can be quite frightening, and when health care providers are rushed, they don't help with your anxiety. It is often very difficult to interrupt a health care provider when they are rushed, and it may leave you feeling lost and confused. There are always other members of the team who can help you find the information you need. Ask for help or for someone else to explain things.

Despite the rather rushed introduction to her treatment from the specialist, Barbara found that the treatments were really not that bad. She got to know the radiation therapists, most of them really young to her eyes, and they were caring and concerned. The treatments themselves were only ten minutes long, and Barbara was able to organize them for the early part of the afternoon on most weeks. She was really tired, and she found it difficult to get up early in the morning. She mostly took taxis to the cancer center and found that she needed to nap most afternoons when she returned to Joan's apartment after her treatment. Joan was so kind to her through the weeks of treatment. She looked after Barbara so well, making her light meals and endless cups of tea. Nothing was too much trouble for her. She even did her laundry, much to Barbara's embarrassment. She was so tired, a tiredness that seemed to come from the depths of her being. She'd also developed some burning of the skin over her abdomen, and this made bathing painful.

Fatigue is a common side effect of radiation treatment, and other than resting and napping, there is really not much that can be done about it. It really helps if there is someone to help you with the usual activities of daily living, like cooking and cleaning and doing laundry.

Skin damage over the area where the radiation passes through the body is another common side effect of this kind of treatment. The skin damage is like a sunburn, and the fairer your skin, the more likely it is that you will have some burning. The nurses and radiation therapists will give advice about how best to care for your skin.

The four weeks of treatment were finally over. Barbara had not gone back to her home at all, and although she was very grateful for Joan's hospitality, she really wanted to be back in her own little house. She went home one Sunday, still really tired but grateful that the worst was over. It was almost three months since her surgery, and spring had arrived. She was eager to get back to her gardening and her old life. What she did not anticipate was that the fatigue did not leave her. It hardly ever got better. Every day was a struggle. She could hardly get out of bed, and like a baby, she had a nap in the middle of the morning and then in the afternoon again. The days were longer and warmer, but she hardly got any of her usual work in the garden done. She looked at her seed catalogs with sad eyes. She had missed the late winter order deadline while she was in Chicago, and the day she had gone to the garden store she had been too exhausted to buy much. She mostly stayed at home, and when her neighbor Sue offered to do her grocery shopping, she gratefully accepted. She still had a lot of food frozen from after her surgery, and she picked at that. Her appetite seemed to have vanished along with her energy.

———⊗———

One of the most common side effects of radiation therapy is fatigue, and it can be severe, preventing the person from doing any of the activities that he or she enjoys or must do. There is no timetable for recovery from this, and many people get really frustrated when the tiredness drags on for weeks or months.

———⊗———

One month after her radiation treatments were over, Barbara was so despondent about the tiredness that she called Irene, the nurse at the cancer center. Irene was sympathetic but could only offer her hope, not much else.

"It can take a really long time to get over the effects of radiation," she explained. "Some people are hardly bothered by fatigue, and others, like you, have a really difficult time of it. Just rest as much as you can, and see if it improves. I think you're coming back to see Dr. Bloom in a month or so, right? I'm sure you'll feel better by then."

But she didn't. The fatigue never left her. It sat on her chest, heavy and pressing, like a bad dream that wouldn't go away. The summer days came and went, and she just stared out the window at her perennials burning in the sun and the empty flowerbeds, the dark earth cracked and barren. It took all her willpower to get on the train to Chicago for her next appointment with Dr. Bloom. Joan met her at the train station, and they went straight to the cancer center.

This time they hardly had to wait at all. Dr. Bloom seemed much more relaxed, and she spent about twenty minutes with Barbara. She seemed a little perplexed by Barbara's complaints of fatigue, and she reassured her that it would improve. Barbara was less hopeful. While they were still talking, Irene entered the room. She listened as Dr. Bloom wound up the interview and then sat down to talk to Barbara.

"The fatigue is still there, then?" she asked, her voice sympathetic.

"I can hardly take care of myself," Barbara replied, her voice even sounding tired. "I've not done anything since I got home, and I'm getting really frustrated with myself. Is there anything that can be done?"

Irene thought for a moment or two and then made a suggestion. "I think a visit to one of our occupational therapists might be helpful. You live outside the city, right? Let me see if one of them is available right now to see you. I'll go and call."

Barbara sat back in her chair, exhausted. But at least Irene had heard her complaints and had not just patronized her. Irene returned about five minutes later. The occupational therapist could see Barbara in about thirty minutes. Irene walked Barbara and Joan to the part of the cancer center where the occupational therapist had her office. Barbara thanked the nurse for helping.

"You don't have to thank me. I'm just doing my job. I know how hard this can be, and I'm happy to be of even a little assistance. Now just sit here, and Cathy will be out to get you. Good luck, Barbara. I'll be thinking of you!"

The two women sat and waited. Barbara fell asleep after a few minutes and was awakened by the sound of her name being called. She struggled to get out of her chair, helped by Joan who told her not to rush. The voice calling her name belonged to a woman in her thirties who came toward them with her hand outstretched.

"Ms. Mason? Pleased to meet you. I'm Cathy, Cathy Anderson, one of the occupational therapists here. Come on in to my office where we can talk. I'm sorry you had to wait for me, but I'm glad I was able to meet with you this afternoon." She turned to Joan: "And you are?"

"I'm Joan, a friend of Barbara's. I can wait outside here if you want."

"Please come with me," Barbara said. "You can tell Cathy how bad this is."

"It sounds like you doubt I'll believe what you say! But your friend is welcome to join us if you want. My office is just down this hallway."

Once they were all seated in Cathy's office, a bright room with colorful artwork on the walls and plants on every surface, Cathy invited Barbara to tell her story. Barbara liked the way Cathy said that: "Tell me your story." She started slowly. She described how tired she felt and how she hadn't been able to do any gardening. She talked about how even after being asleep the whole night she woke exhausted. Cathy asked a lot of questions, and some of them seemed to make no sense to Barbara.

"No, I don't think I'm depressed! Frustrated maybe, but not depressed. Why do you ask that?"

Cathy explained that depression can sometimes be mistaken for fatigue, and the other way around. Barbara thought about it for a moment and then nodded her head. "I remember that one of the teachers I worked with was depressed, and she always complained about being tired. But I really don't think I'm depressed."

"And you may not be, Barbara. I just have to ask these questions to get a better picture of what is happening to you and how I can help you." Cathy continued her assessment. "How do you sleep at night?"

"Well, okay I think, but I'm tired when I wake up, and I'm usually a real morning person."

Sleep quality can affect energy levels during the day. Getting a good night's sleep can really help, but the converse is true, too. Poor sleep is a significant contributor to fatigue. Some strategies that have been shown to improve sleep are avoiding late-afternoon or long naps; limiting time in bed to actual sleeping instead of watching TV in bed before sleep; going to bed only when sleepy; setting a consistent time for going to sleep and waking up; avoiding caffeine, sodas, and other stimulants in the evening; and establishing a presleep routine that is practiced consistently.

Cathy continued her questioning: "Are you getting any exercise?"

Barbara burst out laughing. "You're kidding me, right? How on earth can I exercise when I can barely take care of myself?"

"I know it sounds strange, but exercise can really help increase your energy levels. Before all of this, what kind of exercise did you do on a regular basis?"

"Well, in the summer I garden, and that keeps me in good shape. In the winter I walk when I can. I don't have a gym membership or anything, and it's difficult when it's really cold."

"I know. It's always a challenge. Let's talk about what you can do that will help."

Joan interrupted. "Isn't there a pill or something she can take? It just seems a bit harsh to make someone who's exhausted exercise."

"Yes, it does sound contradictory," replied Cathy. "There have been some studies done with medication with mixed results, but I think it's always best to start with something we know will work rather than using medications that can have side effects. That's just my approach to this, and if Barbara doesn't agree, she doesn't have to follow my suggestions. I can send her back to her primary care provider who may be willing to prescribe something."

There has been a fair amount of study into managing cancer-related fatigue. Some interventions have been shown to work, while others have yet to prove their effectiveness. Exercise is the only intervention that has been shown in studies to help with cancer-related fatigue.

*Here are some interventions that may be helpful: Screen for causes of the fa-
tigue, and manage them as appropriate. Encouraging patients to conserve energy
and alter their activities to manage fatigue may also be helpful. Balancing rest and
activity can help, but the person may have to ask others to help with this, and not
everyone has that kind of support or is willing to ask for it. Relaxation exercises,
massage, and healing touch may also help, although there is less evidence that these
are effective.*

*There have been some studies investigating the use of medication to treat
cancer-related fatigue. The medications tested were mostly stimulants or antidepressants, and although they were helpful for some people, they also had significant
side effects, and experts suggest that the risks may outweigh the benefits.*

"I don't want to take medication," Barbara said quite forcefully. "I'd
rather try this exercise. What exactly would I have to do?"

*Exercise helps in many different ways to improve your quality of life and level
of functioning. It can help lower your risk of heart disease and osteoporosis, improve
balance, lower your risk for depression and anxiety, help with weight control, improve sleep, and combat fatigue.*

*It is important to do the kind of exercise that you enjoy and to customize it
so that you can do it with comfort and without compromising your safety. Some
people really like to go to the gym and work up a good sweat. This may not be possible soon after completing treatments that have left you weak and perhaps with
some challenges keeping your balance. You may need the help of a specialist such as
a physiotherapist or an exercise trainer to help you modify your exercise routine.*

Cathy had a pile of books sitting on her desk, and she looked through
them until she found one that she handed to Barbara. She explained that the
book had some good information about exercise and diet. She also said that
she would be happy to refer Barbara to an exercise specialist, but she would
have to come into the city for that. Barbara refused. She was exhausted from
the day she had spent in the cancer center and just wanted to go home and
rest. She still had to get through the train ride home, and all she could think
of was her bed in her own house.

The two women left the occupational therapy department, Barbara
with guarded hope and Joan with skepticism. A lot of what Cathy said made
sense to Barbara. She had put on some weight since the surgery, and most of
her clothes were tight. She really didn't want to have to buy a new wardrobe
now, and perhaps the exercise would help her drop some pounds.

"I wonder if gardening counts as exercise," Barbara thought out loud.

"Maybe. I've seen you in that garden of yours, and you sure were red in the face after hauling all those plants and bags of dirt! Maybe the book will tell you what to do."

For Barbara, who loves gardening, the good news is that gardening can be a good form of exercise. However, she needs to be careful to stay safe. Perhaps pushing a heavy wheelbarrow will not be possible at first, but over time she can work her way up from watering the garden to pulling weeds to digging. Slow and steady should be the mantra. No matter what exercise you do, you should be able to talk in full sentences without getting short of breath. If you cannot do that, your intensity is too high, and you need to slow down.

Barbara tried to read the book on the train, but she had to fight to keep her eyes open. They just kept closing, and eventually she gave up and let herself fall into a nap as the train moved along. She was startled when the train came to a stop and she realized she was home. She hastily gathered her things and almost left the book Cathy had given her on the seat next to where she'd been sitting.

Later that evening, she picked up the book again and started to read. She found the information very helpful, especially the part about customizing the exercise activity to suit her interests and fitness level. And gardening was a form of exercise, too! She thought about what else she could do. Perhaps she could walk around the track at the high school. That would be fun, and perhaps she'd even see some of the teachers and students. The book suggested that she keep a log of her activity, and she liked that too. She could track her progress, and that would be motivation to continue.

Getting started with an exercise plan is just the first step. It is much harder to keep at it, and there are three simple steps that will help you stick to your plan. The first is to set realistic goals. The second is to reward yourself when you are consistent in actually doing whatever exercise you have planned. And the third is to establish a support system that will validate what you are doing and support you in your plan.

A realistic goal is important because you will only succeed if you can actually do what you have planned. Attempting to do too much will result in frustration and will use up energy instead of creating energy for you. Rewarding yourself is important too, because a reward provides motivation to continue and be persistent. A reward can be anything that feels like a treat: a nice bar of soap that you would not usually buy, a new best-seller, or a movie rental. Having a support system, a person or group of people who encourages you and helps you achieve your exercise goals, can go a long way toward ensuring that you keep up with your plans and goals. Someone who exercises with you can be really helpful, because on any day that you are thinking about not exercising, knowing that you are letting someone else down can be a powerful motivation to just do it!

———❦———

As Barbara left the train station and began walking home, she saw Emily Brown coming out of the grocery store. Emily was one of the teachers at the school, and they had been quite close while Barbara had still been teaching. They had seen less of each other since Barbara retired, but they had an easy friendship with lots in common. Emily waved at Barbara and crossed the street to talk to her.

"Barbara, my dear! I've been meaning to come and visit you, but you know how it is."

"I certainly do. Too much to do, and no time to do it in. How are you, Emily?"

"Oh, I'm fine. Tell me how *you* are. I've been past your house a couple of times this summer, and your poor garden . . ."

"Yes, my poor garden is one of the side effects of the cancer treatment. I've been just too tired to do anything about it, and it looks awful."

"I wish I'd known you needed help," replied Emily. "I would have been happy to lend a hand. The summer's almost over, but are you up to putting in some bulbs perhaps?"

Barbara's spirits lifted with the thought of tulips and daffodils in the spring. "Funny you should mention that. I've been instructed to get some exercise to help with this darn fatigue. And gardening is a form of exercise! So, thank you, I'm going to accept your offer. I'm sure I can manage putting in some bulbs, and it will make spring something to look forward to."

Emily had a broad smile on her face, "Old Doc Doyle told me that I either have to lose some weight or go on pills for my blood pressure. Maybe we could be walking buddies. Do you think you could manage that?"

"I could certainly try. But I have to be careful not to overdo things. I have this book that has information about exercise after treatment. I still need to read it, but I am sure we can figure something out."

And they did figure things out. At first they walked three times a week and for only thirty minutes at a time. Barbara was worried that she would hold Emily back, but Emily was happy to stay at her pace. They talked and talked as they walked around the track on the high school grounds. Summer was over, and the trees were starting to turn color. Barbara loved this time of year, and the temperature was perfect for walking. She had bought a book especially for keeping a log of her exercise routine, and in the last column she wrote comments about how she felt while exercising. When she reviewed her progress, she was pleased to see that all of her comments were positive. She was actually enjoying herself!

One weekend they didn't go on their usual walk and instead spent the days planting bulbs. It felt so good to be scrabbling around in the dirt, and Barbara noticed that she was able to do more than she had originally thought. She sat in the grass on a cushion and gently placed the bulbs in the holes that Emily made with a special planter on a stick. It felt so good to push the dirt over each bulb and pat down the earth. Her neighbor Sue noticed the activity and brought over some lemonade and her special sugar cookies. Emily and Barbara both initially refused the cookies but then took two each, smiling with pleasure as they bit into the sugary crust.

"I've noticed the two of you walking around the track at school." Sue had been successful in her application for the teacher's assistant job at the school. "You two are showing the rest of us up!"

"Well, you have Emily to blame," replied Barbara. "She was the one who suggested it to me. I feel so much better since we started. And look, my pants aren't tight anymore!"

"Hey, it's Barbara who's kept me at it. I only suggested it because I was having some problems with my blood pressure. And I feel better, too! I've lost three pounds since we started, and it hardly feels like an effort."

"Hmm, perhaps I should join you. I have to watch my weight, too, now that I'm having a baby." Sue had a small smile on her face. She hadn't told anyone about the pregnancy, and she hadn't meant to tell the two women, but in the moment it felt right.

Barbara threw her arms around the young woman who had been such a good neighbor to her. "Congratulations! Oh, this is wonderful news! A baby on the street! Will you let me babysit?"

"Of course! I hadn't really thought about that, but it would be perfect, if you still want to when the baby gets here. You don't know what kind of baby I'll have. Maybe you won't want to if he's a screamer."

"I'm sure he or she will be just lovely. You will be a super mom, and your baby will be sweet and kind, just like you."

The three women stood in the fading autumn light, their voices rising and falling with hope and excitement. Spring was going to be a wonderful time with flowers and a new baby. There was a lot to look forward to.

· 6 ·

Where Did That Feeling Go?

$\mathcal{S}$ex and relationship changes are a common challenge after cancer treatment. It is usually at this time that survivors start to think about being sexual again. In this chapter, you will meet Karen and her husband Gary. Karen had a stem cell transplant to treat her leukemia, and she went into menopause with negative consequences for her and Gary's sexual relationship.

Karen was thirty-five years old when she was diagnosed with acute myeloid leukemia. She'd had what she thought was a flu that she just couldn't shake. A visit to her doctor three weeks later led to a blood test and an early-morning phone call the next day telling her to go to the hospital immediately. The rest was a vortex of terror and pain. She stayed in the hospital for eight weeks that first admission and then went home weak as a kitten. Her mother had flown in to help her husband Gary take care of their nine-year-old daughter Emma. Karen was lucky that her sister Joan was a good match and had donated stem cells for a transplant that saved Karen's life. She spent the next year at home, first recuperating and then recovering from the treatment. Her mom Barb stayed on to help. She and Karen had always been close, but the year that Barb gave to her daughter drew them even closer.

Thirteen months after her diagnosis, she went back to work as a lawyer. If someone had told her before her cancer that she would be able to leave her work for that long, she would have laughed at them. But she had to do it, and even though it was harder and harder as the months after the transplant went by, she didn't go back to work. The doctors had warned her about the risk of infection from being in public, and she had listened and stayed away. Then the day came for her to go back, and she dressed in her office clothes, got in the car, and drove to the office. It felt normal and yet strange at the same time. The legal assistants and secretaries had decorated her office with balloons and flowers, and her two partners, friends from law school, had brought in a lovely breakfast. It felt like she was home, and even though she was exhausted at the end of the day, she felt useful again.

Going back to work really did make her feel like a normal person. She had always loved her work as a real estate lawyer, and she slipped back into the daily routine quickly. Her last visit to the oncologist had been a happy one, with her counts all in the normal range. She was in remission, and she was cautiously hopeful. Her mother had offered to stay just a little longer— "to help Emma with the transition," she said—and Karen found herself very grateful for her continued presence. Emma loved having her darling Baba around, and they had grown even closer over the past year. Even Gary didn't seem to mind his mother-in-law being around. He was a litigator in a large law practice, a partner in fact, and the demands of his work could be all-consuming at times. With Barbara there, he was able to continue working through Karen's illness, and he was grateful to her for that.

One night after dinner, Emma and her grandmother went to a movie, and Gary and Karen were alone. They'd opened a bottle of red wine with dinner, and Karen felt a little tipsy. Instead of going to his study after dinner as he usually did, Gary sat down next to her on the couch.

"Hey honey, seeing that we're alone, how about we . . . you know."

Karen was a little surprised. It had been so long since he had approached her in that way that she was not sure what to say.

"Um, well, okay, I guess."

He looked so crestfallen with her reply that she tried again.

"I didn't mean it to sound like that. It's just that it's been so long, and well, I haven't really thought about it."

"Well, you hardly ever thought about it, even before. It's just that it's been a really long time, and I've missed it, you know?"

"Of course I know. I'm sorry, Gary. Really, I am. And my mom and Emma won't be back for a while, so come on, let's see if we still remember."

He laughed as he stood up and pulled her off the couch. Karen tried to smile back at him, but she was too nervous. What would it be like? It had been so long since she had even thought about sex, and she really didn't feel like it now. But Gary was her husband, and she owed it to him. He had always wanted it more than she did, and at times in their marriage it had been a source of conflict between them. She decided to just get it over and done with. She had to try at some point, and this seemed to be as good a time as any. Well, not really. She was exhausted tonight, but then she was exhausted every night. She forced herself to smile at him, and she allowed him to put his arms around her from behind, and they walked in tandem toward their bedroom.

It is not unusual for couples to have different levels of desire for sex. It is usu-
ally assumed that the man has a greater sex drive than the woman, but this is not
always so. It is very common for both men and women to lose interest in sex as
part of the cancer experience. From diagnosis through treatment, sex may disap-
pear altogether as the person faces multiple diagnostic tests and various treatments.
However, some couples find that being sexual provides a welcome relief from stress,
and they may actually be more sexual in the face of a life-threatening illness.

Many people do not feel any interest in sex while undergoing chemotherapy. It
is important to check with a health care provider if precautions need to be taken to
prevent chemotherapy agents from affecting a partner if body fluids are exchanged.
It is often necessary to use condoms to prevent the partner from coming in contact
with semen or vaginal secretions that may contain by-products of the chemotherapy.
For people who have depressed immune systems due to chemotherapy, it may be best
to avoid sexual contact altogether to reduce the risk of infection.

It was a complete disaster. Karen could sense Gary's need, and so she
hurried her own arousal. In truth, she was hardly aroused at all, and so she
pretended she was ready for him to enter her. When he did, she was shocked
at how much it hurt. She felt her whole body stiffen in response to the knife-
like pain she felt in her vagina. She tried her hardest to not make a sound,
to not let the scream she felt behind her eyes come out of her mouth. Gary
didn't seem to notice anything, and within just a few moments it was over.
She lay in the same position, her legs stiff and her arms at her sides. Gary was
breathing heavily, and he moved to his side of the bed and draped his arm
over her stomach. Unable to help it, she jumped out of bed and stumbled to
the bathroom.

"Honey, are you okay?" His voice trailed her as she closed the door
behind herself. It felt like she was broken inside, and she didn't want him to
see her face.

She stayed in the bathroom for a long time, wishing he would fall asleep.
She sat on the toilet, her legs shaking. She tried to pass urine, and the first
drops stung like acid. When she wiped herself, she was not surprised to see
blood on the tissue. She was broken inside! She was not sure how long she
stayed there, but eventually the bright lights made her eyes burn. She opened
the bathroom door quietly, and as she had hoped, Gary was fast asleep. She
tiptoed out of the bedroom.

She sat in the den in her robe, waiting for her mother and Emma to
come home. She sat like that, her robe pulled tight around her, for some
time. Her head was full of thoughts and noise and eventually silence. She
was startled by the sound of the front door opening. They were back from the

movie. Karen quickly wiped her face with her hands, not sure if she'd been crying but not wanting them to see that anything was wrong. They came into the house giggling and whispering. The movie had been good, and they'd had a great time together.

"Karen, you're up! We're a bit late because we stopped for ice cream on the way home. I hope you weren't worried."

"Mom! It was the most amazing movie EVER!" Emma talked in uppercase letters these days, a sure sign that puberty was on its way.

"I'm glad, sweetie. And ice cream, too, to make it even better! How about you go right up and brush your teeth. Say goodnight to your grandmother, and thank her for a lovely evening. I'll be up to tuck you in."

"You don't need to tell me to thank Baba. I already did. With kisses! And you don't need to tuck me in bed. I'm not a baby anymore!"

Karen and her mother looked at each other. Emma was growing up so fast! She sounded like a teenager already, and she was only nine years old! Karen saw sympathy and recognition and memory in her mother's eyes. She'd gone through it, and now her daughter had to, as well.

"Mom, I want to ask you something." There was something in Karen's voice that made Barbara sit down on the couch next to her daughter. It sounded serious, and she wanted to be in hugging reach if that was what she needed.

"This is really embarrassing and I'm sorry to drag you into this but, well, Gary and I made love tonight, and it really hurt. Should it?"

Barbara cleared her throat, trying to buy herself some time. Before she'd married, before Karen was born, she'd been a nurse. She hadn't worked for almost forty years, but she had always been the go-to person for all of Karen's friends when they were growing up. She was not sure what she was going to say, but she also knew that it had taken courage and desperation for her daughter to talk to her about this.

"Oh, honey, I'm so sorry! I thought that by now . . . well, never mind. I know that after I went through menopause, sex just wasn't the same. Your poor dad, well, he just had to get used to it. You've been through a lot, honey, and Gary may just have to control himself."

Karen felt her face flush. Why had she asked her mom? She felt stupid, and that was not something she felt very often.

"Uh, thanks, Mom. For everything."

Chemotherapy often puts women into an early menopause, and some women never see the return of their normal menstrual cycle. The ovaries shut down and stop producing hormones, resulting in hot flashes and vaginal atrophy, as well as a dry and painful vagina. Estrogen is a female hormone that, among other things, keeps the tissues of the vagina moist and healthy. It is sometimes called the hormone of arousal because of its effects on vaginal lubrication.

Many women find vaginal penetration painful after menopause, and it may be even more difficult for women who go into instant menopause from chemotherapy instead of the gradual decline in hormones experienced during natural menopause.

She got up, wincing at the sharp pain that flared between her legs. Somewhere in the first few weeks of chemotherapy, her period had disappeared. Just like that. One month she had it, and then never again. She'd read about that somewhere in the piles of pamphlets they'd given her to read while she lay in the hospital. She was too sick and too weak to do anything else, and now, months later, she had little recall of what she'd read. She'd had lots of hot flashes, too, but those seemed to be getting less and less severe. And now this: a dry vagina. She suddenly felt very old and very tired.

Gary was awake now and in his study, his back to the door, his whole body focused on the computer monitor. Karen stopped for an instant outside the door, but he didn't hear her or he decided not to respond to her presence. His hair was standing up in the back, and for a moment she wanted to go over to him and push it down. But then she might have to talk to him, to explain why she had stayed in the bathroom, or worse still, to answer when he asked if she had enjoyed it. She walked quietly to their bedroom, glancing in at Emma who was reading in her bed, her hair glowing in the soft light from her bedside lamp.

The next morning, she got up before Gary, who must have come to bed very late. She hadn't heard him, although she didn't feel like she had slept very well. She left a note for her mother, with a reminder that Emma was going to play at her best friend Lilly's after school. She drove to her office so deep in thought that when she got there she couldn't remember anything of the drive. Her desk was piled high with files to review, and soon Karen found herself immersed in her work. The hours flew by, and she skipped lunch, hoping to get out early. But one of her most important clients called with an urgent matter, and it was close to six o'clock when she finally got into her car and drove home.

She hadn't eaten all day, and she was hungry. The smell of roasting chicken made her mouth water when she came through the kitchen door.

"That smells amazing, Mom! Is it almost ready? I'm starving. I didn't see Gary's car. Did he call?"

"He's going to be a bit late. He said to start without him, and he'll eat leftovers when he gets home. Emma's ready for dinner—she was asking for cookies earlier, and I told her not to ruin her appetite."

The three women ate dinner together. Karen was tired and quiet, but Emma and her grandmother talked around her silence. The chicken was delicious, and her mom had roasted some vegetables under the bird. They were golden and juicy and slick with chicken fat. Karen started to clean up, but her mother shooed her out of the kitchen.

"Rest, honey. You look like you had a busy day. I can take care of this. Why don't you have a nice bath and then watch some TV with Emma?"

She did as she was told, enjoying the feeling of being taken care of and, yes, even being told what to do. It was a relief, actually, a sharp contrast to her professional day where she had to make decision after decision. Having her mother tell her what to do made her feel younger in a way, and it was easy just to do what she was told.

And that became her pattern. She came home from work, and her mom had made dinner. They didn't talk about how long Barbara was going to stay, and the days blended into weeks. Gary often stayed at work late. In fact it was the exception when he came home in time to eat with the rest of them. Most nights Karen was asleep before he came home. She felt the weight of his body as he lay down beside her, but neither of them touched the other. He went in to work on the weekends too, but she didn't say anything about it. Emma asked where he was once or twice, but then she just accepted his absence. She was busy with her friends, and besides, her grandmother was always there even if her parents weren't.

It can be surprisingly easy to slip into the habit of not talking and not touching one's spouse or partner. And that leads to a gradual drifting apart until the couple lives like college roommates. While some couples are happy to live in a sexless relationship, lack of sex can lead to a lack of emotional closeness, as well as sexual frustration. It can be quite difficult to change this pattern, and as the days and weeks and months go by, the distance makes it even more difficult to start a conversation about what is happening to the relationship. Some couples find themselves arguing more, while others don't even engage in that way and just drift further and further apart.

On Gary's birthday, he came home from work early, and they went to a steakhouse to celebrate. Emma and Barbara had made a chocolate cake. It was slightly lopsided because Emma didn't fill the cake pans equally and she overdid the frosting, but it was a lovely cake. They cut the cake when they came home from the restaurant, and uncharacteristically Gary did not go straight to his study to work. Barbara diplomatically left the den and went to her room to watch TV. It felt a little awkward to Karen, sitting on the couch so close to Gary and yet so far away too. They started to talk about work, and

Karen felt her eyes drooping. She'd had two glasses of wine with dinner, and she was exhausted.

"I think I'm going to bed," she said, getting up from the couch.

"No use in me joining you, is there?" was his sharp reply.

"What does that mean?" she bristled, knowing full well what he meant but wanting him to say it out loud.

"Well, it's not like there's any point to me being there with you, is there? You somehow manage to avoid me at every opportunity, Karen. You're either asleep when I get home, or you're gone in the morning before I get out of the shower."

"You're one to talk! You're hardly ever home. Emma has even stopped asking for you. You seem to be deliberately avoiding me!"

The fight continued well into the night. They'd both had enough wine to shorten their tempers and sharpen their tongues. The fight went round and round, accusations followed by recriminations, and eventually they went to bed, too exhausted to argue anymore but with things far from resolved.

It is said that couples argue over three things—money, in-laws, and sex. Sexual problems can be the spark for much bitterness because sex represents different things to different people. Either partner can see lack of sex as personal rejection, and this can hurt very deeply. It is also possible that one person may assume things that are not true. However, if they don't talk about it, these assumptions become an insurmountable barrier because the other person may not even know what the original assumptions were.

Things continued like this for another three weeks—Gary stayed at work late, and then when he was home, they argued. Barbara pretended for a while that she didn't hear their heated words, and she tried to ignore the obvious tension when they were in the same room. But one day she said something to Karen after a night when they had argued until close to 1:00 a.m.

"I don't like to interfere, but the two of you had best get some help for what is going on. I haven't heard either of you say a civil word to each other in weeks, and Emma asked me yesterday if you two are getting a divorce. You need to fix this before it really affects that girl. It's not fair to any of you. Get some help!"

Her words stung, especially the part about Emma asking if they were getting a divorce. That weekend, she told Gary that they needed to see a marital therapist. She didn't really know where the words came from, and she was surprised when he agreed. She looked in the Yellow Pages for a counselor located near their offices downtown and made an appointment for them to see her the following week.

The first session did not go well. Gary was distracted and silent and hardly said a word. The therapist asked a lot of questions, and Karen felt like she was the only one answering. They argued again that night at home. They were both lawyers and were used to using their words to encircle and trap, so once again it was thrust and parry, attack and counterattack, with no resolution. The next week they had a return appointment with the therapist, and Gary didn't show up at the appointed time. Karen sat there waiting for him, embarrassed and angry and confused. Didn't he want to work on this?

Marital therapy or couple's counseling can be an effective way to resolve differences and get the couple talking to one another in a meaningful way. The counselor or therapist can control the conversation and prompt positive ways of resolving conflict. But both partners have to engage in the process, and when one withholds or refuses to participate, it can be difficult.

She sat silently in the waiting room of the therapist's office. "This is useless," she thought and left the office. She remembered to leave a check for the appointment but refused the therapist's offer to reschedule.

"My husband obviously doesn't want to work on this, so it would just be a waste of your time and my money. I'm sorry."

She walked back to her office feeling defeated. Perhaps there was nothing to save in their marriage. They had drifted so far apart in the past few months that she was not sure they could find each other again. She thought about the horrible days following her diagnosis and how strong he was and how he had helped her. She didn't remember much from that first admission to the hospital, but he had been there for her and now he was gone.

In the shock after hearing the words, "You have cancer," most couples report that they have never been closer. The crisis forces people to consider what they have and what might be lost, and this is often affirming for the relationship. But that intensity may be harder to maintain in the long term, and it is not uncommon in the months and years after cancer treatment for couples to reassess their relationship, and sometimes one of the partners may be found wanting.

The experience of cancer may precipitate the breakup of a relationship that no longer meets the needs of the person with cancer. Sometimes people feel that after everything they have been through, they no longer want to be in a relationship that is troubled or that is lacking in something that is important to them. And there are times when partners of cancer survivors end a relationship because they just can't do what is demanded of them.

Later that week, Karen had a routine appointment with her family physician. Julie Barker was her primary care physician but also her friend. They knew each other from college and had an easy friendship. They were both so busy in their professional lives that these days they only saw each other when Karen had an appointment or occasionally at a fund-raising benefit. Karen was looking forward to the appointment in a way. They hadn't seen each other in what seemed like a long time. She usually booked the last appointment of the day so that she and Julie could chat after the official part of the appointment.

"Hi, friend!" Julie Barker burst into the room with her usual energetic stride. "I haven't seen you for ages. How are you?"

To both of their surprise, Karen burst into tears in response to the question. "Whoa!" she spluttered when she eventually managed to stop crying. "I didn't expect that to happen. It's just . . ."

And then for twenty minutes she told her friend and physician everything. She hardly stopped to take a breath, and the words poured out of her. Julie sat and listened, her face creased in concentration and concern. When Karen stopped, Julie took a deep breath and then started to speak.

"You've been through a lot, Karen, and I'm sad to hear that it's not over. As you probably know, chemo can put you into premature menopause, and that's often worse than when you go through it naturally. Would you be interested in taking hormones that would help?"

Karen hesitated. "I don't think I want to do that. I just don't feel right putting something artificial in my body like that. I'm not even sure that I could, with the cancer and everything. But let me think about it for a while. I'll get back to you on that."

Dr. Barker nodded. Her head was still full of the information that Karen had told her. It sounded like her marriage was in trouble, real trouble, but she didn't know Gary all that well, and she wasn't sure what she should do about that part.

In recent years, hormone therapy for women after menopause has received a lot of attention in the media. A large study was published in 2002 that suggested that hormone therapy did not prevent cardiac disease in women and in fact was harmful. As a result of that, millions of women abruptly stopped taking hormones, and many experienced significant side effects from stopping the medication suddenly. Further information on the use of hormones during menopause has received less attention. The suggestion now is that hormone therapy can be used in women with moderate to severe menopausal symptoms, but the lowest dose should be used for the shortest time possible. These hormones should be used only to treat symptoms of menopause such as hot flashes and vaginal dryness and should not be used as prevention for cardiac disease.

———

"I'd best get home," Karen said as she got up from her chair. "My mom has been amazing, but I do need to spend more time with Emma. Gary's hardly at home when she's awake, and I can't let my mom take over everything. I'll see you soon."

When she got home, her mother was putting the finishing touches on dinner. The house smelled of roasted chicken, and there was a large green salad on the table waiting to be tossed.

"Gary called. He won't be here for dinner. Emma's upstairs just finishing up her homework. She wanted to watch something on TV this evening, so she got a head start on that project she's working on. Oh, and I saw something when I was at the library today—I put it on your desk. It's an information session put on by that new women's clinic in the strip mall. I thought you might be interested."

"Thanks, Mom. I'll just put my briefcase down and wash my hands. The chicken smells delicious."

As she put her briefcase on her desk in the study, she glanced at the colorful pamphlet lying in front of her computer monitor. As her mother had said, there was a new women's health clinic at a nearby mall, and they were advertising an informational discussion on menopause for Monday evening. She looked over the pamphlet and then threw it down on the surface of the desk. What could they tell her that she didn't know? Even Julie, her friend and doctor, didn't seem to have much to offer. And what would solve her problem with Gary? Just thinking about Gary made her shoulders tighten, and she could feel the beginnings of a headache at the back of her skull.

They ate dinner, which was as delicious as the smells suggested. Emma chatted about school and the project she was working on, and Karen let her mind drift. She kept thinking about her response to Julie and the pamphlet lying on her desk. It was funny how the two things happened on the same day. Maybe there was a message in that. After dinner, she went back to her study and looked at the pamphlet again. Perhaps she would go to the session. It was just down the road, and she could leave at any time if she didn't find it useful.

The following Monday evening, she found herself sitting in her car outside the clinic. She'd told her mother that she needed to pick up some items at the drugstore, and Barb had waved her off. Emma was putting the finishing touches on her project, which was due the next day, and the two of them had their heads together, checking carefully to make sure it was as perfect as it could be.

The pamphlet said the session started at 7:30, and Karen waited until a few minutes later to enter the clinic. It was brand new, with the smell of paint and carpet in the air. The session was being held in a conference room, and Karen had to stand at the door. There were no empty chairs, and the room was full. She leaned against the wall and listened as a young woman introduced the three speakers who would be talking that evening. One was a physician, one a pharmacist, and the other a sex therapist. They each spoke for about twenty minutes, and Karen felt her mind wandering as the first two speakers talked. The final speaker of the evening was the sex therapist, a woman about her own age with spiky dark hair and long dangly earrings. In a lively voice, she began:

"So you've heard from my colleagues about hot flashes and osteoporosis; and yes, one of them even said the *v* word. Menopause can certainly cause a dry vagina, but what I want to talk about is how that can affect your relationship."

Karen felt her face get hot, and she knew she must be as red as a radish. It was as if this woman was talking directly to her and about her, and she leaned forward from her place against the wall. Some of what the therapist was talking about got lost in her head as her thoughts started to whirl. But snippets of her presentation stuck in her head: she talked about how things can change for a woman during menopause and how this could cause conflict in a relationship. She talked about how medication might solve the physical problems, but how some couples needed help talking about what was happening. And she offered her services to help anyone who wanted some help.

Karen felt as if the room was suddenly brighter. As the audience left after the question period, she stayed behind. She approached the sex therapist—Molly was her name—and asked if she could see her as a patient.

"Of course I can see you! What's your name? Come with me to my office, and I'll see when I next have an open appointment."

She followed Molly down the hallway, and within minutes she had an appointment for Friday afternoon. The clinic was new, Molly explained, so they were not that busy. But she hoped that would change soon, and that was one of the reasons they had decided to hold the information session. Molly walked with her to the door of the clinic and waved as Karen got into her car.

She drove home, barely noticing the other cars on the road. As she walked in the door, she remembered that she'd said she was going to buy something, and yet she didn't return with anything. Oh well, if her mother asked, she would make something up. She started laughing when she realized that she was acting like a teenager. "That's what happens when you lie to your mom," she thought.

Gary wasn't home yet, and her mother and Emma were still fussing over the project.

"I've got some work to do on a file. I'll be in my study. Emma, don't stay up till all hours with that project, okay?"

"Yes, Mom" was the only reply she got.

The week flew by, and soon it was Friday, the day of her appointment with the sex therapist. She left work early and drove to the clinic, suddenly nervous about what they would talk about. She felt a little guilty about seeing the therapist without talking to Gary, but she had hardly seen him all week. And besides, she was here to talk about her own problems, not him.

She didn't have to wait at all and was taken directly into the therapist's office on her arrival.

"Hello, Karen. It's nice to see you again. Come and sit down over here and we'll get started. Now, what has brought you here today?"

Karen was not sure exactly where to begin. She told Molly about the leukemia and the stem cell transplant. She described how tired she was and how helpful her mother had been.

"Okay, thanks for sharing that, Karen. But I'm a sex therapist, and I need to know what it is that brought you to see me and not the physician or any other member of our team here."

"Well, it's just that . . ."

"I know it's difficult to talk about for most people. But there's nothing you can say that I haven't heard before. Perhaps it'll be easier if I ask you some questions. How about you tell me how your sex life has been since your cancer treatment?"

"Well, there's only been the once, and it hurt like anything. I even bled a little bit, and since then there's been nothing."

Once she started talking about it, she was surprised how easy it was to continue. Molly was a good listener, and Karen found herself talking about things she hadn't even realized were important to her. Molly prompted her with questions every now and then. "What's happening between you and your partner with all of this?" "What have you tried to help the situation?" "What do you think about medical treatment for this?"

A skilled therapist or counselor can usually elicit a lot of information with carefully worded questions. Often the person has not thought about the problem from all angles, and this skillful questioning can provide the person with solutions that come from within. The therapist can help you find your own answers, and this is often more useful than being told what to do.

After Karen talked for some time, the therapist made a suggestion. "It sounds to me like you think this is *your* problem that only you can solve. This is a couple's issue, Karen, and you will only solve this if your husband is involved. You need to bring him with you to our next appointment. But there are some things that I would like you to consider before that. There are some options for you that will help with the physical symptoms you describe. The first is hormones."

Karen opened her mouth to stop the therapist.

"Just let me continue. There are a range of options, and medication is just one of them. There are also a number of vaginal moisturizers and lubricants that can provide some relief. These are just options, and my suggestion is that you try a number of them. I have some samples that I can give you to try. Let me put them in a bag for you with some written information. Read it, and try these products. And the next time we meet, we can talk about whether any of them were useful. Does that sound like a plan?"

Karen nodded. The session had been exhausting, and she just wanted to get out of there. How was she going to tell Gary about this? She knew he would be angry that she had gone behind his back, but he had hardly been around to tell him. She left the clinic feeling distracted and nervous. The small plastic bag in her hand felt like it would explode, and she tossed it on the passenger seat of the car. What was she going to tell Gary?

She waited until the weekend to talk to him. He usually slept a little later on the weekend, and instead of going off to run errands as she normally did, she hung around the house, waiting for him to get up. He stumbled into the kitchen just after nine, his hair standing up in clumps and his face covered in stubble. She was sitting at the table, absently reading the newspaper. She'd made coffee and had placed his mug on the countertop close by.

"Morning," he mumbled, squinting at her. "How come you're still here? Don't you do something on Saturday mornings?"

"I wanted to talk to you, Gary. But not here. Emma will be up soon and my mom . . ."

"Sounds serious. Are you okay? Did you go to the doctor?"

Gary's usual way of dealing with anything he was not sure of was to go into lawyer mode and fire off a string of questions. That was actually the way he dealt with most things.

"There's nothing wrong. Well, nothing to do with the cancer. Well, that's not true either. Gary, I just want you to listen to me and not say a word until I'm done, okay?"

He nodded, his face now creased with concern. He rubbed his hand over his jaw, another sign that he was confused and unsure of what was happening.

"Ever since my treatment, I've been in menopause. You knew that, right? Well, do you remember the last time we made love? Well, I didn't tell you, and I don't know why, but it really hurt, and I had some bleeding after that. It's been really hard for me to talk about this. Anyway, I went to this talk on menopause at this new women's clinic at the mall, and they have this counselor on staff, so I made an appointment to see her. And, well, she wants to see us together. She wants to see you, I mean."

Karen eventually paused to take in a breath. Gary took the opportunity to start asking questions, but she held up her hand to stop him.

"I'm not done. I know you're mad, and I know I should have told you all of this before. But you haven't been around much, and I just didn't know where to start. I thought . . . I hoped I could sort this out myself, but Molly, the counselor, said that this is a couple's issue, and she wants you to come to my next session with her. Okay, now you can talk, but please don't yell. I don't want Emma to hear us fighting again. Mom said that Emma asked her if we're getting a divorce."

Gary's voice was clipped and just louder than a whisper. "Why am I the last person to know *anything* in this house?" His voice was getting louder, and Karen reached out her hand to him, but he moved away, and his chair clattered to the floor.

"Gary! Please! Don't wake Emma! Let's go outside on the deck. Or in the car. Just please don't yell!"

He stormed out of the house, the back door swinging shut and almost clipping her shoulder as she rushed to catch up with him. Her car was in the garage, and he threw open the door, climbing in on the passenger side. The plastic bag with the samples from the sex therapist lay on the seat, and he picked it up as he sat down. Karen suddenly had a thought.

"Open that and take a look inside. There's some stuff in there from the counselor."

He upended the bag, and the samples of lubricant fell into his lap.

"What the . . . ? What is this? What is all this stuff?"

"I got this from the counselor at the clinic. It's some samples of stuff that she thought might help. I haven't looked at it yet. She thought it might help with the dryness."

"Karen, you'd better start from the beginning. Who is this 'counselor,' and why does she need to see me? What kind of counselor is she?"

Karen took a deep breath and told him everything. He sat silent, staring out of the car window at the garage wall as he listened. He was furious that she had not talked to him about any of this, but he had to admit to himself that his response over the past months had been to work longer hours and to avoid the tension in the house.

"Okay, I'll go with you. But I am not interested in any funny nonsense, you understand? What exactly does a sex therapist do anyway?"

Some people are not sure what a sex therapist actually does, and there are many misconceptions about sex therapy in general. A sex therapist is a highly educated professional who is usually certified, most often by the American Association of Sex Educators, Counselors and Therapists (www.AASECT.org). Sex therapists may specialize in one particular area (for example, working with couples who are dealing with chronic illness) or may see a wide range of couples and single people who are experiencing sexual difficulties. Sex therapy usually involves talking about the problem and figuring out what might help. It does not *involve nudity or having sex in front of the counselor.*

After the weekend, Karen called Molly and made an appointment for late the following Friday afternoon. Gary made a bit of a fuss because it meant he had to leave work early, but one look at Karen's face and he didn't say anything more. Karen remembered that Molly had told her at her first appointment to try the product samples, so she pulled the plastic bag out of her bedside drawer late one evening. She stared at the samples. What were they for? She couldn't remember what Molly had told her, and she wasn't sure what to do with them. She read the pamphlets that were in the bag. One described how to use the various moisturizers and lubricants, but she was still confused. She opened one of the sample packs and was surprised when a clear gel-like liquid slipped out and into her hand. It was very slippery, and she looked around for a Kleenex to wipe her hand on. There was nothing close at hand, so she went into the bathroom to wash her hands. When she came out, Gary was sitting on the bed, reading the pamphlet she had left lying there.

"This makes it all sound so, I don't know, clinical. What is all this stuff?"

"It's just some samples that Molly gave me to try. I opened one package, and it was kind of goopy. I'm not really sure what the differences are between them all, to tell you the truth."

"Well, how about we give one a try?"

Karen stood very still. Did he mean he wanted to have sex? She immediately felt her throat tighten, but then she thought about it for a minute. Perhaps they could try. The last time had been months ago now. She hesitated, and Gary jumped up, his face getting red.

"Well, sorry I even suggested it. You'd think I would learn my lesson."

"Gary, hang on. It's not that. It's just that it's been so long, and the last time hurt. But I miss you and the closeness we once had. I really do! Let's just try, okay? We can use one of these lubricants, and maybe that will help."

So they tried. They opened one of the sample packages, and it made a little difference. Karen was really tense, but it did hurt less. At least she didn't feel so dry. Once again it was over really quickly, but this time Karen didn't run to the bathroom. She lay next to her husband and listened as his breathing got slower. When she was sure he was asleep, she got out of bed very quietly and went into the bathroom. There was no blood this time, but she felt tender down there. Would she ever enjoy sex again, she wondered?

There are a large number of lubricants and vaginal moisturizers available, many of them at your local drugstore. They are not, however, interchangeable. Vaginal moisturizers are used to keep the vagina feeling comfortable; they are not used to make penetrative sex more comfortable. These moisturizers should be used three to four times per week (following the instructions in the package), and then less often to maintain comfort. Replens and Liquibeads are vaginal moisturizers.

Lubricants are used for sexual purposes. There are even more of these on the market, and it is important to read the ingredient labels. Water-based lubricants are the most common type sold in drugstores, and most people would recognize K-Y Jelly, which is water based. It tends to dry out quickly. Astroglide is another water-based lubricant that contains glycerin. Some women find that this causes yeast infections. Other water-based lubricants are Embrace and Frixxion. Astroglide now comes in a new formula without glycerin or parabens that may be less irritating. Other lubricants without glycerin are Maximus, Liquid Silk, Oh My (claims to be organic), Probe, and Slippery Stuff. These are available online and through sex stores.

Products that are silicone based (look for dimethicone in the ingredients list) stay slippery for much longer but can only be removed with soap and water. Be careful when using these in the bathroom, as they can cause falls. If the silicone lube gets on the floor and you step in it, you will go for a nasty spill. Some silicone lubricants are Eros, Wet Platinum, and Pink.

Some people prefer natural oils, and these can be effective as lubricants. But they are not safe to use with condoms as they destroy latex. Olive oil, almond oil, or coconut oil may be used. Basically anything that is edible is safe to put on or in the body. For more information about lubricants, see chapter 12.

Friday afternoon came quickly. Karen was nervous about Gary not showing up at the appointment. But they talked about it the night before, and he said he would be there. And he was. They both pulled into the parking lot at the same time, and although he looked nervous, she knew that she probably did too. She was not sure what to expect at the appointment with Gary there. Would it be different than when she was on her own? How would Gary react to Molly's questions? When she thought about it, Molly hadn't asked her many questions, just one or two, and then she had listened to her, really listened to her. Maybe that's what she would do with Gary, too. As they walked toward the door of the clinic, she reached out and took Gary's hand. It was big and strong and warm, and in that instant she realized how much she'd missed holding his hand. It had been a long time since they had done that too.

Molly was standing behind the reception desk when they came through the door, and she took them into her office immediately. Karen could feel the tension in Gary's body as he sat down on the couch next to her, and she once again took his hand in hers.

"So, here you are!" Molly had a warm smile, and Gary's shoulders relaxed just a little. "I know that this can be scary, but I want you to know that nothing will happen here that you are not in agreement with. My role here is to help you identify how you can help yourselves get back to the way you used to be or to find a new way for you to be as a couple. How does that sound?"

"What do you mean by that?" Gary had kicked into lawyer mode, and Karen patted his hand.

Molly tried again. "So, Gary, what has it been like for you since Karen's diagnosis and treatment?"

"You mean in the sex department?"

"You can start wherever you like. What has it been like for you?"

And just like Karen had the week before, Gary started to talk. Karen sat in shock and listened as he described how lonely he had felt, how isolated, and how terrified he was of losing her. As he talked, he stared at the wall, not looking at either Karen or Molly. Gary had always been good with words. It was one of his great skills as a litigator. But he had never used his words like this before, and Karen felt the tears come to her eyes as she listened to his pain. Molly asked a few probing questions, and he talked even more. This time he looked at Karen as he spoke, and she held her breath as the words entered her heart.

"Honey, it's just been so hard to not be able to be with you physically. It was always so good for us, and then after your treatment, it just ended. We didn't talk about it. It just was gone. We've never been one of those lovey-dovey couples, but the sex was always amazing. And then there was, well, nothing."

Molly interrupted. "What has sex meant to you, Gary?"

"Well, everything. No, I don't mean it like that. The sex was always great. And she seemed to like it. Didn't you?"

Karen couldn't answer. There were tears running down her face, and her throat was so tight that she couldn't get the words past the constriction. She nodded.

"So sex was the way you expressed your love for her, and when that went away, you had no other way." Molly repeated what Gary had said.

"I guess so. I just didn't know *why* it had gone away. I mean, I saw how sick she was with the transplant, but then you went back to work and I thought that things would go back to normal. I had no idea what was going on. We just stopped touching, and that was that."

"Our time is almost up, I'm afraid, but I'm going to make a few suggestions. It's common after someone has gone through an acute illness like this for things to change. And it can be difficult for couples to get back to where they used to be sexually."

Karen interrupted the counselor. "But we made love the other night. We used one of those samples you gave me, and it was better, much better."

"I'm going to suggest something that may sound radical. For the next six weeks, I want you to try something called sensate-focus exercises. It's a tried-and-true way for couples to find their way back to each other. I have printed instructions here for you that explain it in detail. This is the radical part—while you go through this exercise, penetrative sex is forbidden, at least for the first four weeks."

Karen and Gary stared at her. What had she just said?

—∞∞—

One of the most useful couple-oriented activities for enhancing mutual sexual enjoyment is a series of touching exercises called sensate focus. Masters and Johnson, the famous sex therapists, labeled this technique and have used it as a basic step in treating sexual problems. It can be helpful in reducing anxiety caused by goal orientation and in increasing communication, pleasure, and closeness. It is a very useful technique for people after cancer treatment, as it allows for a gradual return to sexual activity when the couple is unsure about what is possible to do and what might be different.

In the sensate-focus touching exercises, which are done two to three times a week, partners take turns touching each other while following some essential guidelines (see chapter 12 for a detailed description).

—∞∞—

"I thought this was supposed to be sex therapy, not 'no sex' therapy!" Gary attempted to make a joke.

"Ironic, isn't it?" Molly replied.

She'd heard this many times before, and she knew that for many couples it could be a struggle. They wanted to fix things quickly, to go back to the way things were before. But cancer changed everything, and for some couples, things are never the way they were before—not better, not worse, just different.

"So, I'd like to see you back here in about two weeks, after you've given these exercises a good try. It's going to take commitment and discipline and time. And I know that time is always a problem."

"We'll make the time, won't we honey?"

It was Gary who spoke, and this surprised Karen a little. How were they going to make the time? His answer to her unspoken question came from his firm grip on her hand. He was going to try; they were going to try.

· 7 ·

Feeling Fit

*T*reatment for cancer can ravage the body, and it is important to eat well and exercise to regain strength and heal the body. Morrie had gone through bladder cancer, and Esther, his wife, decided they were going to turn over a new leaf. She began to cook differently and insisted that they exercise every day. What did Morrie think about this?

Esther and Morrie have been married for forty-two years. They have three adult children and four grandchildren who live within walking distance. Theirs is a home of laughter and love as well as really good food. Esther has a community-wide reputation as an excellent cook. Morrie has been the beneficiary of this cooking for forty-two years, and it shows in his girth. At five feet six inches tall, he is almost as wide as he is tall. His children have always bugged him about his weight, and now the grandchildren have joined in. He laughs at them when they tell him to go on a diet. And he ignores them when they encourage him to go for a walk or get some other form of exercise. He is a happy man who loves food and good Scotch, and he is not interested in anything getting in the way of that.

One thing that he does do is see his physician every year for a checkup. Both of his parents died when he was young, and somehow he thinks this yearly visit will prevent his early death. His physician is a family friend, and between checking his blood pressure and listening to his heart, the two men joke and talk about their mutual friends. At sixty-six years of age and despite his weight, Morrie has been very healthy—no blood pressure problems, no diabetes, just slightly raised cholesterol, which he blames on Esther and her cooking, not his eating. His doctor keeps telling him he is a lucky man, and he believes him.

This year at his checkup, everything seemed normal. He had to give a urine specimen, and he joked with the doctor's assistant that his urine looked better than champagne in the specimen jar. She laughed at his joke. Every year he made the same joke, just changing the kind of liquid—apple juice, Chardonnay, and now champagne. He went home and told Esther that he was good for another forty years, and she was happy to hear that he was well. She worried about him, but then she worried about everyone in her family. She was the pessimist, and he was the optimist. The children always said that they balanced one another perfectly.

Three days later, Esther answered the phone and was a little surprised when the caller identified herself as Dr. Rosen's assistant and asked for Morrie. Esther's heart immediately skipped a beat. What was wrong? The woman wouldn't tell her anything and left a message for Morrie to call the office. Esther called Morrie on his cell phone, and of course he didn't answer. He turned his phone off most of the time despite her nagging that he needed to be available if she called. So she waited and waited for him to come home. He was at the community center with his chess buddies. They played chess once a week, and he was usually gone until the early afternoon. The minutes ticked by so slowly, and when he eventually walked into the house just before three o'clock, she was furious.

"Where have you been? I've been trying your cell phone over and over!"

"You know I don't like to be disturbed when I'm playing chess. It takes all my focus to beat those useless old men I play with!"

"Enough about chess! You have to call Dr. Rosen. Someone called from there this morning, and she wouldn't tell me what it was about."

"Don't worry your lovely head about it. It's probably just someone to tell me what a miracle I am. Sixty-six years old, and I have the blood pressure of a twenty-two year old!"

Esther glared at him, and with a shrug he went into the spare room to make the phone call. She hovered outside the door, trying to hear what he was saying, but he was hardly talking, and her heart sank. When he came out of the room, he almost bumped into her.

"What is it? What's wrong?" were the first words out of her mouth.

"It's nothing, nothing. Dr. Rosen just wants to take another look at me. There was a little something in my urine."

"Oh no! What are we going to do? It's bad, I know it's bad."

Esther started to cry, her usual response to anything that bothered her. And as usual Morrie tried to calm her down. His nature was not to worry about things until he knew for sure what he was dealing with, and hers was the exact opposite. They had been through some crises in their forty-two years together, and he knew that with time she would calm down. He reassured her that he was going to see Dr. Rosen the next day, that the doctor would take care of things, and he pleaded with her not to tell the children anything, at least not yet.

The next day he went to see Dr. Rosen, who explained that there was some blood in his urine, a tiny amount that was seen when the sample he had given was examined under the microscope. Dr. Rosen believed that patients needed to know the truth about everything, and so he admitted to Morrie that he was concerned it could be bladder cancer. Morrie just nodded his head. That was his suspicion, too.

Bladder cancer occurs more frequently in men and may be diagnosed on the basis of the following symptoms: blood in the urine that may be visible to the eye or only seen under a microscope, frequent or painful urination, and abdominal or back pain. It is usually diagnosed early and treated successfully. A definitive diagnosis is usually made after additional testing, which may include a cystoscope (an examination of the inside of the bladder with a special instrument that is passed through the urethra and into the bladder), a biopsy of tissue from the bladder, a CT scan of the organs of the urinary system, and a special imaging test called a pyelogram.

The next few days for Morrie were filled with tests and doctor's appointments. He had to tell Esther what was going on, but he pleaded with her not to tell the children until they knew something for sure. He knew this was difficult for her, but he didn't want to worry anyone. He knew that Esther was filled with worry, and he could see that she was trying her best to be strong, but he heard her crying in the bathroom. Even with his optimistic outlook, he was also worried, but he tried to put on a brave face for her.

On a sunny Monday afternoon, he and Esther both went to see Dr. Rosen to hear the results of all the tests. Dr. Rosen was quite serious when he sat down at his desk. It was bladder cancer, a transitional cell carcinoma, which is the most common type of bladder cancer found in North America. There was good news, too. The cancer was just in the lining of the bladder and had not invaded the bladder wall. Morrie would not need surgery and instead would have immunotherapy, where medication would be instilled into his bladder. This medication would prompt Morrie's own immune system to fight the cancer cells. It was a lot to take in, and they both left the doctor's office with thoughts swirling in their heads.

They told their children about the cancer the next weekend. As expected, they were very upset, and Morrie had a difficult time persuading them that it was not the end of the world. They were used to him downplaying the seriousness of almost everything, so this time they thought he was fudging the truth about how serious the cancer was. It was only when their father went to call Dr. Rosen at his home that they settled down. Morrie could see the worry in their eyes as they left with their own children, and he was both touched and also a little irritated. He knew he was going to be fine! Why wouldn't they listen to him?

Morrie saw the cancer specialist and started the treatments later that week. It wasn't so bad, just a bit uncomfortable when they put the catheter into his bladder. He had to have a treatment every week for six weeks, and the doctor told him that any side effects would be mild. Easy for him to say, thought Morrie after the second treatment, when he felt like he had to urinate every thirty minutes throughout the night. He moved into the spare bedroom so as not to disturb Esther, and she was not pleased with him. They had hardly ever been separated for all the years of their marriage, and she liked his warm bulk beside her at night. It was really just the night and the day following the treatment when he felt any different.

—⚬⚬⚬—

Cancer of the bladder is treated according to the stage of the cancer. If the cancer has not invaded the wall of the bladder, it is often treated locally with the installation of medication directly into the bladder. If the cancer has gone into the bladder wall, surgery is usually required.

—⚬⚬⚬—

The six weeks of treatment went by fast. Esther fussed over him, and Morrie actually enjoyed the extra attention. They had told most of their friends about his cancer, and the wives brought cookies and pies every week, gifts of love for their dear friends. There was nothing Morrie loved more than baked goods, and he indulged often. After the first three weeks, Esther started telling their friends not to bring anything to the house, but the containers kept coming. Esther put some of the food in the freezer, and she gave some to their children, but there always seemed to be a plate or a pie dish on the kitchen counter. She didn't have a sweet tooth herself and could pass on the treats, but Morrie nibbled away at whatever was available. She knew in her heart that this was not good for her husband, but she felt powerless to stop him. He always did just exactly what he wanted to do. He didn't listen to her and would make a joke out of it if she was insistent on something.

She went with Morrie to see Dr. Rosen after his last treatment. The doctor was pleased at how well Morrie had tolerated the treatments. He told them that the cancer specialist had suggested that Morrie have a yearly examination of his bladder and also yearly installations of the medication into his bladder for about five years. Morrie already knew this. The cancer specialist had given him a number of documents with instructions about what would happen next, but it was good to hear that Dr. Rosen was in the loop too.

"So, Morrie, did you actually read all the material you were given?"

"Well, almost, Doc" was Morrie's reply.

"He never does what he's told," interjected Esther. "You know what he's like. He reads a bit of this and a bit of that, and if he doesn't like what he sees, then he puts it away. I, however, have read everything!"

Dr. Rosen smiled. He loved observing the interactions between his older patients. And when the patient was someone he had known over the years, their conversations were just so much more interesting. There was so much love between Esther and Morrie. His parents were good friends of the couple, and he felt honored to be Morrie's physician.

"So, Morrie, did you read the part about eating properly and getting some exercise?"

Without skipping a beat, Morrie replied, "Oh, no, Doc, there was nothing in the papers about that! Just some stuff about seeing my doctor and having more tests every year."

Dr. Rosen didn't have to say anything. He knew that Esther was going to jump right in. And she did.

"Morrie—what nonsense you talk! Of course there was something in there about that! But like I said, when he doesn't like what he sees, he just ignores it. It's the same when I tell him something. He just ignores me. It's like I never said anything!"

"Morrie, I've been telling you for some years now that you need to lose some weight."

Dr. Rosen had hardly spoken the words when Morrie interrupted him. "But Doc, look at me—perfect blood pressure, no diabetes. You said so yourself when I was here for my last checkup. I'm a miracle!"

"You're a lucky man, Morrie. But your luck won't hold out forever. You're also significantly overweight, and that can cause other problems for you. Many people like you find that being diagnosed with cancer is a wakeup call, and they make some important lifestyle changes."

"Oh, Doc, you told me that the bladder cancer was not so bad."

"I told you that you had stage 1 bladder cancer and that you were lucky that we caught it early. It's still cancer, Morrie, and you're not out of the woods yet."

"You tell me what he has to do, and I will make sure he does it." Esther's voice trembled just a little bit. She loved her husband, but she also knew him well, and if she didn't do something, he would just laugh it off. This cancer had scared her, and she was worried that he wasn't taking it seriously.

"Well, for a start, your husband needs to start eating better. And he must get exercise, regular exercise. Both of these will help him to lose weight. He needs to lose a lot of weight, both for his heart and for his cancer."

"Hang on a minute here, Doc!" Morrie's face was red, and his voice was loud. "What does my weight have to do with the cancer?"

―⁂―

There is increasing evidence that obesity and cancer are linked, although the precise nature of the link is not clear. Obesity has been shown to adversely affect a cancer prognosis, so it is very important that anyone with a cancer diagnosis maintain a healthy weight for his or her height. In addition, obesity causes many other health problems such as diabetes and heart disease, and these remain significant threats to overall health and well-being outside of the risks of cancer. Other risks to health come from smoking, drinking alcohol, and a lack of physical activity.

―⁂―

Dr. Rosen walked over to a filing cabinet and started searching for something. While his back was turned to the couple, Esther shot a stern look at her husband. He smiled at her and reached out his hand, but she just crossed her arms. She was mad at him, and he knew it. And this time his sweet smile was not going to make her feel any better.

Dr. Rosen finally found something, a pamphlet as well as a sheet of paper. He smiled in apology. "This is not much, but it will give you something to start with. I was sure I had more for you, but I just can't seem to lay my hands on anything else."

"That's okay, Dr. Rosen. I'm sure the kids can help us find more information on the Internet." Esther was now eager to get out of the doctor's office. She had a job to do now, and she wanted to get started as soon as possible. Morrie might think this was a joke, but she didn't, and she was going to get their children and grandchildren involved. They left the doctor's office. Morrie was still trying to get her to smile at him, but she was determined not to give in to him this time. This was a serious situation, and she was not going to make a joke out of it, no matter how hard he tried.

When they got home, there were some messages on the answering machine. They were from their sons and daughter as well as their two daughters-in-law. Their eldest son, Jeffrey, was a lawyer, and his wife Shelly was a nurse. Esther intended to get some help from her. Their next child was their only daughter, Susan, and Esther knew that she would be a valuable asset because she was Morrie's favorite. And the youngest was Bernie, their son who taught mathematics at the university. His wife, Bonnie, was very close to Esther and would help out in any way she could.

Esther waited until Morrie was settled in his favorite armchair, the remote control for the TV in his hand, his attention focused on finding something to watch. She called all three of her children's houses. Susan was home, and they spoke for a while. She then left messages for Shelly and Bonnie. She asked them all to meet her that weekend at Susan's house, and she also asked them not to say anything to Morrie about the meeting. She told them that there was nothing to worry about, but she needed their help. And she wanted the men there too. She was not sure what she was going to do when she met with them, but she knew that she would have a plan by then.

Shelly, Jeffrey's wife who was a nurse, called the moment she got home and heard the message from Esther.

"Esther, is everything okay? Is Morrie okay? You sounded worried in your message."

"We're fine, nothing to worry about. We just saw Dr. Rosen, and he wants Morrie to lose some weight. And of course that foolish old man treats this like a joke. So I thought that I could get you kids to help me with him."

"Oh, that's great! Thank goodness that's all it is. I'm not working this weekend, but Jeffrey has this big trial coming up, and I'm sure he's going in to the office most of the weekend."

"Maybe before that, if you have time, you could look into what kind of diet he should be on. Dr. Rosen gave me a pamphlet, but it doesn't have much information."

"I'll talk to one of the dieticians at the hospital. I'm not sure if there's anything special for someone with bladder cancer, but she should know."

Esther smiled as she heard these words. Shelly was a real go-getter, and if anyone could find useful information, it was she. She worked in the intensive care unit at the university hospital, and even though Esther didn't understand exactly what she did, she had a lot of experience and knew a lot about all sorts of health stuff.

Esther met with her children and their spouses on Saturday afternoon while Morrie went to get his hair cut. Even though Jeffrey had planned on working on the trial all weekend, he really wanted to be part of the discussion, so he stayed home and worked there. They were all concerned about why their mother had called this family meeting, fearing that something bad had happened to their father. Esther reassured them that, as far as the doctors knew, Morrie had responded well to the treatment, and he would have regular testing to watch for any recurrence. What she was concerned about, and what she needed their help with, was his weight and general health.

She was a little surprised when her two sons admitted that they were also very worried about their father's weight. Jeffrey, the lawyer, had lost almost twenty pounds the previous year after he had started running. Bernie, the professor, had always been thin, but he had started yoga some time ago and had also become a vegetarian. Susan had two small children at home, and she only bought organic foods. They were all very supportive of any initiative to help their mother and ultimately their beloved father.

"I talked to one of the dieticians at the hospital," Shelly offered. "She said that she isn't an expert on cancer, but she gave me some books. I read through them quickly, and there do seem to be some important modifications that Morrie can make in his diet."

"So tell me—what should I know?" Esther took out a pen and some paper and sat waiting to take notes.

"There are some general things he can do, and there are also some very specific things. What kind of detail do you want?"

"Everything!"

Although what you eat won't cure cancer, a good diet may help you stay healthy and can help you regain strength, fight infection, and feel better. It is important to eat a varied diet with a focus on plant-based foods. Colorful fruits and vegetables contain the most nutrients. Whole grains and legumes are good sources of complex carbohydrates and fiber. Consume less than one cup of lean protein and low-fat dairy products a day. Minimize your intake of fat, salt, sugar, alcohol, and smoked or pickled foods. Steam, boil, or poach your foods instead of frying or charbroiling.

Esther scribbled down every word as Shelly read from a book in her lap. Bernie and Jeffrey nodded as they heard confirmation of what they had been doing. Susan was leafing through another book, and she interjected, "There's all sorts of stuff here about nutrient-rich foods. Maybe that's what we all should be doing—go organic, and eat these super foods."

Shelly looked up. "Maybe Esther should see a nutritionist about the specifics before she changes their diet so radically."

Esther sensed the tension in her daughter-in-law's words. Shelly and Susan had butted heads before, and she didn't want them to fight. "I will see a nutritionist; it's an excellent idea. But what else does that book say, Susan?"

"Well, it says that organic is better than the regular stuff, which is why I only buy organic, and also that these super foods contain all sorts of things that can help."

There is evidence that nutrient-rich foods do contain vitamins, minerals, fiber, antioxidants, and phytochemicals that can help you stay healthy, but they do not influence the development of cancer or its recurrence. The following have been identified as nutrient-rich foods: berries, Brazil nuts, citrus fruits, colorful vegetables, and also cruciferous vegetables such as broccoli and kale. Moderate intake (up to six ounces, two to three times a week) of fish such as wild salmon, sardines, black cod, and striped bass is also recommended, and it is better to eat wild fish than farm raised. Flaxseed and legumes, such as lentils, beans, and peas, provide valuable fiber in the diet. Cooked tomatoes provide a valuable source of antioxidants, and yogurt with live cultures can help keep the immune system healthy. Black, green, and white tea are also recommended instead of coffee or soda.

———————

Esther was still writing down the information, struggling a bit to keep up with what Susan was reading. In frustration, she put down her pen. "I can't write this all down! You read too quickly!"

"Then stop writing and just listen, Mom." Jeffrey was always the logical one. "If you're going to see the nutritionist, which I think is a great idea, I'm sure she will give you all sorts of books and lists and things. Let's talk about how we can help you and Dad."

"Well, maybe you can support me when I tell him not to eat something and he just ignores me. You know how he gets, especially when there's cake or cookies around."

"Maybe we can get him to exercise, too," suggested Bernie, who had always been the jock of the family despite his nerdy appearance. As kids, they used to joke that he was like Clark Kent, bookish on the outside and Superman on the inside.

"Ha! I'd like to see that!" was Jeffrey's cynical response.

"Well, you turned yourself around, so why couldn't Dad?" Susan had always been a daddy's girl, and she hated it when anyone criticized her father. "Maybe if we took turns going for walks with him."

"I'd like to do that." This time Bonnie jumped into the conversation. She was a librarian at the university where Bernie taught mathematics, and she usually kept to herself, finding the rest of the family a bit overwhelming, perhaps. "Maybe we could even get the kids involved. I know Emma would love to spend some time with her grandfather."

Bernie and Bonnie had one child, a shy six year old named Emma. Like her mother, she too found the rest of the clan very noisy. Jeffrey and Shelly had one daughter, a bright and beautiful sixteen year old named Lilly who was training to be a singer. Everywhere she went there was music, either coming out of her headphones, which she seemed to wear constantly, or out of her mouth as she hummed and sometimes sang scales. Susan's two children, Simon and Jason, were rambunctious boys who constantly yelled and fought with each other. Susan was separated from her husband, and since he moved out almost a year ago, the boys seemed even noisier. Jeffrey and Bernie thought Susan had lost control of her kids but were too afraid to say anything. She was a bit fragile, and they didn't want to upset her.

"That's a wonderful idea!" Esther was pleased that they all seemed to want to help. "I know your Dad would like nothing more than to spend time with his children and grandchildren. Maybe we can make a timetable."

Making lifestyle changes, such as improving diet and increasing exercise, can make a significant difference in the quality of life for cancer survivors, especially those who are older and overweight. Cancer can be a wake-up call, not only for the person with cancer, but also for their family members and friends. But making these lifestyle changes is not easy. It requires motivation and commitment, which can be difficult to sustain over the long term.

Survivors who believe that an unhealthy lifestyle (smoking, alcohol consumption, unhealthy diet, or lack of exercise) contributed to their diagnosis of cancer are more likely to correct the unhealthy behavior. And survivors who believe that a healthy lifestyle can prevent recurrence are also more likely to make changes in their lifestyle.

As much as Jeffrey wanted to be part of this, the thought of the work he had to do in preparation for the trial was at the forefront of his mind. He needed to get back to his files and preparation, so he tried to take charge.

"Okay, so do we have a plan here? I hear that we should all be encouraging Dad to get some exercise and also that Mom is going to go to the nutritionist. What else do we need to do right now?"

"Oh for goodness' sake, Jeffrey!" Shelly could see how her husband wanted to get back to his work. "Why don't you just leave, and the rest of us will continue the discussion. But don't think you're done with your part! You'll be walking with your dad, and you'll have other responsibilities, too."

Jeffrey almost bolted from the room, stopping briefly to kiss his mother on the top of her head. As the door closed behind him, they all sat in silence for a few minutes. This is how things always went with Jeffrey. He was the oldest of the siblings, and somehow his needs and desires always came first. And Esther always covered for him.

"Just let him go. You know how worried he is about the trial. And I need to be going, too. Morrie will be back soon, and I don't want him to know about this."

"How can he not know about this?" Bernie was getting irritated. As the youngest, he really looked up to his father, and he was feeling increasingly uncomfortable that they were all talking about the man when he was not there. "Mom, when you go to the nutritionist, Dad must go with you. You can't expect the man to make these changes in his life without being part of the decision."

"He's right, Esther," Shelly said, and both Bonnie and Susan nodded their heads in agreement. "This won't work without his cooperation. He needs to be in on this every step of the way. Ultimately it's his life, and you can't fool him into eating differently or getting more exercise."

"I know, I know, but he's such a stubborn old man! You all know that!"

"But Mom, he loves us—you, especially—and he wants to be around to see his grandchildren grow up. If we can explain it that way, maybe he'll be more willing to make the changes."

Not only is it challenging to make lifestyle changes, but it is even more difficult to sustain them in the long term. People need all the help and support they can get, and having a loving and involved family is a definite asset. Studies show that cancer survivors do make lifestyle changes. In one large study, almost 92 percent of survivors did not smoke, and almost half got regular exercise, but less than 20 percent ate the recommended five servings of fruit and vegetables a day. Only 5 percent of cancer survivors in this study met all three recommendations.

The next day, Shelly arranged for Esther and Morrie to meet with the nutritionist at her hospital at the end of the week. Esther had talked to him about the meeting she had with their children, and to her surprise, he was upset that she had kept it a secret from him.

"This is *me* you're talking about! Don't talk about me behind my back! Not even to my children, especially not to my children!"

And so the two of them went to the appointment with the nutritionist. She was a young woman with dark hair and a broad smile. She spent almost two hours with them, starting with an assessment of Morrie's diet. She laughed when Esther kept correcting her husband, reminding him that most of what he ate he didn't put on a plate but moved it from the serving plate to his mouth.

"You sound like so many other couples I've met. Many of us eat unconsciously, and that can add up to a lot of extra calories—often poor calories, too. I have some simple strategies to help with that."

"Is there some pill I can take? In case I don't eat so healthy all the time?" Morrie was not 100 percent convinced that this new diet was going to work.

"That's a great question. Most people find it difficult to get all their essential nutrients from food. So, yes, a good, balanced multivitamin is a good idea. But read the label. Some products contain more than 100 percent of your daily requirements, and that is not a good thing. Speak to your pharmacist about what brand you should buy. They are knowledgeable and helpful.

And you may need to take additional calcium and vitamin D supplements, too. For a man your age, you need 1,200 milligrams of calcium a day."

"Our daughter Susan thinks we should be eating organic foods only. Is she right?"

"Ah, the organic question!" replied the nutritionist. And then she began to explain.

———

There is no strong evidence that organic food is any more nutritious than other food, but there is a big difference in the way organic food is produced and processed. Organic farmers do not use pesticides for their crops, and their livestock are not given hormones or antibiotics. These products may be healthier for us. However, they are also more expensive and may not be available in smaller towns or cities. Going to a farmer's market may be a good thing to do, but it does not mean that the produce is certified organic. It is important to ask if the products sold by individual farmers have been exposed to chemicals. Organic food also tends to spoil more quickly and so should be bought in small quantities and consumed quickly.

———

"So, Esther, what exactly am I going to be eating for the rest of my life?" Morrie had listened to everything the nutritionist had said, but he needed a picture of it in his head to truly understand the changes he was going to be experiencing. Esther looked up at the nutritionist, hoping that she would answer Morrie's question. But the nutritionist merely nodded at her, indicating that she should answer.

"Okay, let me look at my notes for a minute. You're going to be eating less meat and more fish. And much more fruit and vegetables, too. And less fat, we have to cut out the fat. Oh, yes, and whole grains instead of bagels and cookies. What am I missing? Oh, yes, dairy. Only skim milk and no more cream. Did I get it right?"

The nutritionist nodded. "Yes, you did. There is much more detail in the books I am going to give you and some sample menus with recipes and even shopping lists."

———

It is important to eat a varied diet with a few key components. Fruits and vegetables are essential, and the more colorful, the better. Anything that is deep green (spinach and kale for example), red, yellow, or orange (peppers, red apples) contains high-quality nutrients. A serving of fruits and vegetables is half a cup, and cancer survivors should try to get eight to ten servings each day. Whole fruit and vegetables are better than juices. Whole grains are another essential component of a good diet after cancer (as well as for everyone else, too!). You should eat at least three servings of whole grains each day. One serving is a slice of whole grain bread, a half cup of whole grain pasta or rice, or half of a whole grain pita or bagel. It should be easy to see that getting three servings a day can be accomplished quite easily with toast for breakfast and a sandwich for lunch.

Cancer survivors should keep their fat intake low, about 44 to 55 grams a day (or 20 to 25 percent of daily calories). Avoid saturated fats, which are found in animal proteins such as cheese, bacon, sausage, and whole milk. Avoid processed foods such as margarine, salad dressings, and commercial baked goods, as they contain saturated fats and omega-6 fats. Monounsaturated fats (found in olive oil, canola oil, avocados, and nuts) are preferred and can be used to make homemade salad dressings. Be wary of packaged or prepared foods that are labeled "low fat," as they are often not that different from regular food, and always check the serving size—you may be surprised that a serving is much less than what is in the package. Always check the label on any can or package for the presence of trans fats, which are the worst fats of all and should be avoided. Increasingly, trans fats are being banned and used less frequently in commercial products.

Limit your intake of red meat (beef, lamb, and pork) to twice a week at most, and ensure that the portion size is about the size of a pack of playing cards. And always consume only low-fat or nonfat dairy products made with skim milk.

—⊗⊗⊗—

"It's a lot to take in, I know," the nutritionist said reassuringly. "You can always come back to see me if you have more questions or need a refresher."

Esther could sense that her husband was overloaded and wanted to leave. She had a lot to think about, too. They left the nutritionist's office with a bag full of books and pamphlets. Esther knew that these changes were not going to be easy, but she was determined to make them and to bring Morrie along with her. They had a lifetime of eating habits, some of them bad, to modify, and it was going to be a challenge for Morrie to eat more fruits and vegetables, but she wanted this more than anything for him.

When they got home, they were surprised to find Susan and her two boys waiting for them. The boys were both wearing their bike helmets, and they started shouting as soon as they saw Morrie get out of the car.

"Pa, Pa! Come ride with us!"

Laying on the grass just to the side of the path were their two bikes, a two-wheeler with training wheels for Simon, age five, and a tricycle for Jason, who was just three.

"Come with us, Dad," called Susan. "The boys want you to come with them to the park. Come on, it'll be fun! You can help keep an eye on Jason while I help Simon."

Esther smiled. As usual, Susan knew her father so well. He loved those two boys, and he also loved spending time with his daughter. Morrie smiled at his wife and went to help Susan get the boys on their bikes. They pedaled unsteadily down the path, and Esther could hear their voices as they moved down the street toward the park. She went inside slowly, weighed down by the heavy bag with all the information.

Just after supper, Bernie arrived. He had just come back from a yoga class, and his face was shining from exertion. He went to get a glass of water in the kitchen where his mother was putting away the leftovers. He shook his head when she offered him something to eat. He found that it took a while before he could eat after his yoga class, so he declined.

"Where's Dad?" he asked. "I want to talk to him about something."

"He's probably out back, putting the car away. Susan was here with the boys, and Dad went to the park with them. He was quite exhausted when he came back. Those boys are full of energy."

Bernie went looking for his father and found him sitting on a deck chair, his head resting against the canvas. A loud snore escaped his open mouth, and Bernie hesitated before gently waking him.

"Hey Dad, wake up! You know it's not good to nap so close to bedtime. Don't let Mom catch you. You know she'll get mad."

Morrie woke with a start, an embarrassed smile on his face as his eyes adjusted to the dim light.

"Bernie! To what do I owe this honor? Susan and the kids were here today, too. What's going on? Do you know something that I don't? Am I dying and no one will tell me?"

"Oh, Dad, it's not that at all. Well, there is something. Mom told us about what Dr. Rosen said, and . . ."

"Why did she do that?" Morrie was instantly angry. "Why does she have to get you kids involved? I'm dealing with it!"

"Dad, she loves you. We all do. We want you to be around for a long, long time. Don't you want to dance at Emma's wedding?"

Morrie nodded. His anger was dissipating but he was still irritated that his wife had talked to the children.

"Well, you need to lose some weight, and we want to help you. I know you and Mom went to the nutritionist today, and eating healthily will make a difference. But you need to get some exercise, too. And I'd like to help you."

"I'm telling you now that I am *not* going to do this fancy yoga like you!"

"I know that—but maybe you'll change your mind. You should see some of the old guys that come to the class."

"Bernie! I mean it! No yoga. I have no intention of turning myself into a pretzel."

"Okay, okay. No yoga. But maybe you could walk a bit? Maybe do some weights at the community center?"

"I'll think about that, maybe. My friend Steve goes there since his heart attack, and he's looking pretty good for an old guy with a crappy ticker."

———

Recommendations from the American Cancer Society, the Centers for Disease Control and Prevention, the American College of Sports Medicine, and the World Health Organization advise cancer survivors to participate in moderate exercise for thirty minutes or more at least five days a week. Survivors should get the approval of their oncologist before starting an exercise program, and if there is a risk that long-term effects of cancer treatment may affect the cardiovascular system, then assessment and screening should be done first to ensure that the survivor is healthy enough.

Some larger cancer centers have rehabilitation programs where survivors can participate in a managed setting where their overall well-being can be monitored. There are also supervised exercise programs at many community centers, and some focus specifically on people who have had a cardiac event such as a heart attack or stroke.

———

Morrie settled into his new eating regimen with few problems. In the beginning it was new and interesting, and although he joked about eating like a rabbit, he actually enjoyed eating more salads and fresh fruit. There were things that he missed, like cookies and ice cream, but Esther refused to have them in the house. So, unless he sneaked behind her back, his access to them was limited. One night they went to visit friends, and Esther was shocked when she caught him with crumbs all over the front of his sweater. He looked sheepish, and she glared at him. It hadn't been easy for her, either! She had to shop for fresh produce every second day, and there was a lot of washing and chopping involved in making the salads. She didn't speak to him in the car on the way home, and the next day she complained about him to her daughter-in-law Shelly.

"Oh, Esther, everyone makes mistakes! And he's been so good this far! I'm sure that one slipup won't ruin his progress. Maybe you should talk to the nutritionist again and get her opinion on how bad the occasional cheat really is."

Shelly always had good advice, so Esther called the nutritionist immediately. The young woman seemed happy to hear from her, and she laughed when Esther reported that Morrie had been caught with cookie crumbs all over his sweater.

"Everyone cheats at some point," she explained. "Think of it as a 90/10 split. If he can stick to the new plan 90 percent of the time, then he's allowed the occasional treat. How are things going for you?"

Esther told her that Morrie was doing well. He was eating what she made for him, and he even seemed to be enjoying the fresh fruits and vegetables. He had even started exercising!

"That's wonderful!" exclaimed the young woman on the other end of the phone. "What is he doing for exercise?"

Esther described how their children came around two or three times a week and went walking with him. He had even been to the community center to check out what programs they had, and he seemed interested in a swimming program that would be starting at the beginning of the next month. The nutritionist sounded genuinely pleased that Morrie was making these important changes in his life.

"And how about you, Esther? How do you feel about all of this?"

"Funny you should ask. I think I've lost some weight, too. My pants are looser, and that roll of fat around my middle seems smaller."

Although making lifestyle changes may not be easy, it is often more difficult to maintain the changes over the long term. As the novelty of the new behavior wears off, some may find that their commitment decreases, and they slip back into old habits. Family and friends can be great motivators and supporters. It has also been shown that when health care providers encourage their patients to make and sustain lifestyle changes, patients are often highly motivated to follow their suggestions. But it is a long process, one that you should follow for the rest of your life, and the temptation to stop may be quite strong. Including a variety of physical activities may be helpful in preventing boredom, and including some element of socialization, such as exercising with friends or family members, can help, too.

Two months later, Morrie felt like a new man, despite the cancer. He had to admit that he felt better than he had in years. He hadn't weighed himself, but his pants were much looser, and he had to take in his belt two full notches. And it hadn't been that difficult! There was a lot of chewing involved in eating the salads, but they were actually tasty. He didn't really miss the red meat all that much, and now that Esther allowed him the occasional treat, it was fine. He even enjoyed the exercise now that he wasn't so short of breath every time. It was great to walk and talk with his sons on their weekly walks, and spending time with Susan and her boys was the highlight of his week. He wasn't sure that he had to, but pretty soon he was going to tell Esther how grateful he was to her. And he couldn't wait to see her face when he told her.

· 8 ·

What Should I Be Looking For?

$\mathcal{F}$or the cancer survivor, extra attention should be paid to preventing other illnesses, including secondary cancers. One way of ensuring that this happens is to have a survivorship care plan, a carefully laid out document of what to look for, what tests to have, and how often, as well as a detailed description of the treatments the survivor had. Sue's story illustrates this. Treated for leukemia as a teenager, Sue's parents asked the health care team for a detailed summary of future care and monitoring for their daughter. Seven years later, they are still following that plan.

Sue, at age twenty-two, has few signs that she was once a very sick fifteen year old. She was diagnosed with leukemia just days after her fifteenth birthday, and she spent the next two years in and out of the hospital. As an only child, Sue's parents doted on her, and the threat to their only daughter's life changed their outlook on everything. Life changed radically for Sue, too. She went from being a carefree teenager to being a waif-thin child who depended completely on her parents for her every need. But she was one of the lucky ones, and seven years after her diagnosis, she leads a normal life—well, normal for someone who survived a life-threatening cancer diagnosis.

Sue and her parents hardly ever talk about the two years when she was undergoing treatment. It's just too painful for all of them. They also remember different aspects of it. For Sue, it was a time of both physical and emotional pain and confusion; for her parents, it was a terrifying roller coaster of hope and despair. But she went into remission, and since then she has been quite well. She missed a lot of school in the two years of active treatment, but she managed to catch up and was allowed to graduate with her class. But she didn't go to college with her classmates and instead took a year off to rest and

119

recover. A year later, she started taking some classes at her state college, and now at the age of twenty-two she has an arts degree and dreams of becoming a nurse.

———

The survival statistics for childhood cancers has improved dramatically in the past twenty-five years. Where once only 20 percent of children and teenagers survived cancer, now almost 80 percent do, and that number continues to grow. However, these survivors continue to have complex physical and emotional needs.

———

When Sue was in the active phase of treatment, she spent most of her time in the hospital, with the odd discharge home for a week or two, and then she would go back to the hospital. After her treatment was over, she spent months at home, resting and gradually recovering her strength. She saw her health care team frequently during that time, at first weekly and then every second week, and finally every month. She hated going back to the hospital or the cancer center. It reminded her of being sick, and she wanted to feel like a normal person.

She didn't look like a normal person, and being in the hallways and waiting rooms of the cancer center reinforced that. Her face was swollen like a basketball, and her skin was as pale as a sheet of paper. At first she wore a knitted cap to protect her bald head, and then when her hair started to grow back she wore a baseball cap. She saw other teenagers who looked like her, and instead of this making her feel better, she hated the thought of what she must look like to them. For this reason, she avoided her friends from school. This was easy to do. She just said that her doctors had told her that being in crowds was too dangerous for her health. But she was lonely, and she was sure that her parents were tired of her and her needs. She tried not to complain, but she knew that she was irritable and demanding at times, and then she felt guilty.

At the age of twenty-two, she still lives at home and often feels like she is much younger. Her parents have been very protective of her ever since her diagnosis, and at times it was just easier to let them organize her life. She only received her driver's license six months before her last birthday, and she can see how nervous they are when she asks to take the car. She knows *why* this has happened, and most of the time she can live with her parents' involvement in her life. But there are times when she wishes they would back off and let her be twenty-two instead of treating her like she was still fifteen. It's as if her life stopped with her diagnosis, and she has just been stuck there ever since.

———

It is very common for a life-threatening diagnosis to have an effect on the normal developmental stages of a family. The usual milestones and changes are not achieved, and teenagers continue to be treated as helpless children long after they have grown beyond the stage of dependence they were at when the cancer happened.

The developmental tasks of the teenager are to establish strong peer relationships and to begin establishing romantic and sexual attraction to members of that peer group. Teenagers also experience cognitive growth and are increasingly able to think in the abstract and to understand the consequences of their actions. Risk taking is often a central part of teenage experimentation, as is a preoccupation with body image.

Significant illness will have an impact on these developmental tasks. Teenagers have reduced opportunities for social interaction with their peers, and parental control and involvement in activities of daily living prevent independence. Also, the effects of treatment may alter the teenager's physical appearance. As a result, preoccupation with body image may take on an exaggerated nature.

Depending on the kind of cancer and its treatment, some teenagers with cancer experience negative side effects in cognitive functioning and are not able to achieve the expected intellectual and cognitive changes.

Sue knows that she is one of the lucky ones. She has survived the cancer and has managed to go to college. She can think about planning for her future, and she can dream of the day that she will be a nurse and will be able to help others, just like the nurses helped her. She has had few problems since her treatment was over. Her parents have been very supportive and have provided for her financially and emotionally. They have watched over her and made sure that she had the best medical care. They even have a special folder in their home office detailing her complete medical and treatment history. Every blood test or X-ray report has been filed in its place for the past seven years.

At the center of this file is something that her parents call "The Plan." Sue doesn't remember where The Plan came from, only that it came home with her from the cancer center one day, and since then her parents have consulted it regularly. She doesn't remember much from those days, but five years ago, her family was told that she was in remission and that they had to follow The Plan. And they have, even when Sue begged and pleaded with them to let her skip this appointment or that test.

"But Mom, I keep going for these blood tests, and everything is fine! What would be so bad if I skipped it just this once?"

"Now Sue, you are just being silly. The Plan says that you have to have these blood tests every six months with an X-ray every three months. And we abide by The Plan because it's worked for us. Let's not spoil things."

Sue could not argue with her mother. Her mother was like a rock, and it was her determination that had carried Sue through some really difficult times. Her mother's unflinching stance on so many things related to Sue's treatment had become almost mythical in the life story of their family, and so Sue backed down. She was due to enter nursing school in just two months' time, and the summer days flew by.

———∞———

Some cancer centers and oncologists provide patients and their families with something called a survivorship care plan. Details of what is contained in this document are provided later in this chapter. At a minimum, the care plan contains information about the kind of cancer the patient/survivor had as well as the type and duration of treatment. In addition, it might contain information about the kinds of tests the survivor needs to have in the future.

———∞———

And then it was September, and Sue started nursing school. The days were long but exciting, and Sue felt that she was finally in the right place. None of her fellow students knew her history. To them she was just the oldest student in the class; she was not the girl with cancer. It felt good to feel like an adult, not like the perpetual child she was in her family. She liked being a student, and the days and weeks flew by fast. Soon the first semester was over, and then the second. She had a break over the summer and then started the second year, which was much more interesting as they were learning about diseases instead of just anatomy and physiology.

Late in the second semester of her second year, they started a unit on cancer. Sue was surprised by how nervous she was just opening the textbook to the oncology chapter. Would she learn something in there about her own cancer that would shock or scare her? It was as if a new world opened for her in the pages of her textbook. There was so much to learn about! She thought she knew about cancer from her own experience, but in fact she knew very little. She found herself staying behind after class was over and asking the professor many questions.

"Dr. Grant, what about young people with cancer? How does it affect their growth? And what about their families? What impact does the diagnosis have on them?"

"You seem to be really fired up about this topic, Sue," the nursing professor replied. "Has this touched you personally?"

"Umm, I don't like to talk about this, but yes, it has. I was diagnosed with leukemia when I was fifteen."

"Ah, and how are you doing with having to study this? For some students, this can be a real challenge."

"Funny you should say that. I guess I'm realizing that I don't really know much about my own diagnosis and treatment. I mean, it was seven years ago, and I guess I've been pretty passive about it all. My mom, well, my mom took charge when I was in the hospital, and she has been in charge ever since. I just do what she tells me. I go to see my oncologist every year, and that's pretty much it."

"So is that enough for you?" Dr. Grant asked gently. "Do you want to find out more about your own cancer? Or do you just want to leave this alone? Remember that at some point during this semester you will be going on your clinical rotation, and if you want to avoid the oncology unit, just let me know, and we'll be sure to send you somewhere else."

"Oh thanks, Dr. Grant! I don't know what I want to do. But I'll figure it out. I think I need to talk to my mom about this and maybe find out more about my diagnosis and treatment. Can I talk to you next week after class?"

Many survivors don't know the details of their cancer or treatment. For some, this is a way of coping with what happened. For others, it may be because their cancer was diagnosed when they were a child or teenager, and they were not given the information. Still others may have been given the information verbally, and in the busyness of treatment, they have forgotten. Or if they were given something written, they may have lost the documents.

When she got home after class that day, Sue asked her mother about The Plan.

"I guess we should have talked about this before," her mother responded. "But you didn't ask, so I thought you weren't ready. I think it's a good idea that you have a look at it after all this time. It might explain things to you that make more sense now."

Her mother went to the drawer in the office and pulled out a thick folder stuffed with photocopied papers and X-ray reports. Sue looked at it and felt her pulse racing. What would she find? Suddenly she was not sure she wanted to look at whatever was in there, but she took a deep breath and held it in her hands. Her mother sat with her for the next hour as she went through the folder. They didn't talk at all. The only sound in the room was the turning of the pages as Sue methodically read her whole cancer history. At the very back of the folder, in its own envelope, was The Plan.

"Is this it? The Plan?" Sue asked her mother. In her mind, The Plan was something special, and yet in reality it was just another pile of papers.

"Yes, that's what they gave us when we got the news that you were in remission. They told us that everything we needed to know about your follow-up care was in The Plan. And we've followed it to the letter. Can you see where we've checked off things as we completed them?"

Sue looked at the papers again, and there in the margins were small, neat check marks. Every time she'd gone for a blood test or an X-ray, her mom had checked it off. The Plan was a detailed summary of Sue's cancer journey from the very beginning, with instructions for what needed to be done for years after her treatment was over.

———⊗⊗⊗———

What Sue's family refers to as "The Plan" is in essence a survivorship care plan, something that is increasingly being used to help cancer survivors and their families understand their cancer and their ongoing care. There are many different survivorship care plans available. Some are intended to be completed by the health care team and then shared with the survivor's primary care provider as well as the survivor. Others can be completed online by the survivor, assuming that he or she knows the details of the cancer diagnosis and treatment. Some examples are provided in chapter 12.

Although the contents of these care plans differ, they usually contain the following information: the kind of cancer, including stage and grade; a summary of the treatment, including surgery, chemotherapy, radiation, and adjuvant treatment (the amount and dose of drugs and radiation are usually provided); the schedule for follow-up blood tests, X-rays, CT scans, and MRI tests; the schedule for follow-up medical appointments with an appropriate provider (a specialist versus a primary care provider); information about risks to the patient and how to identify signs of recurrence; information about long-term side effects of treatment; recommendations for healthy lifestyle practices, including diet and exercise, smoking cessation, and risk modification; and other resources for the survivor and his or her family.

The survivorship care plan is often presented in paper format but may also be available online. For cancer survivors who were diagnosed and treated as children or teenagers, the survivorship care plan may contain instructions and recommendations about transitioning to an adult care clinic when they reach a predetermined age. The care plan is usually discussed by the oncology care team with the patient (and parents, when appropriate) to ensure that he or she understands the information and has an opportunity to ask questions.

———⊗⊗⊗———

"It's kind of weird to see it all in black and white," Sue said quietly.

"I guess we're so used to it that I really didn't think of it from your point of view," replied her mother. "I personally have found it to be very helpful. In the beginning we were so afraid, and this reassured us that we were doing everything we could, everything that needed to be done to make sure. You know what I mean?"

"Yes, I think I do. I don't remember so much about what happened in the beginning. And then, I haven't really thought much about my follow-up care, either. You were in control of it, and I let you have that control."

Sue's mother interrupted her. "You're twenty-two now. Maybe it's time that you took control of this. How do you feel about that?"

"I don't know, really. Learning about cancer at school has been a little strange. None of the other students know that I have, um, that I had cancer back then. But today I talked about it a little bit with one of my professors."

"You did? Why?"

"Well, I asked her a lot of questions after class. She asked if I'd had an experience with cancer, and I just sort of told her. She asked if I was okay with studying about it. That got me thinking that I hardly know anything about my leukemia, so I wanted to see my file."

"Did looking at The Plan and all the reports help you?"

"I think so. It's a lot to take in, and it's brought back some memories. But I think it's okay."

———

Everyone is different when it comes to knowing about their cancer and the treatments that were given. Some people want and need to know everything, and others don't want detailed information. It's a personal choice and one that should be respected by the health care team. It is very common for the parents of a child or teenager with cancer to control the amount of information given to their child. But with time, and as the child or teenager grows older, it is usually appropriate for that person to know more about the cancer and its treatment.

As discussed earlier in this chapter, cancer can have an impact on the normal maturation of a child or teenager. Sometimes it may be difficult for the parents to let go and allow children or teenagers to act their age, even when they become young adults. They may try, often unconsciously, to protect their child, and in doing so they don't allow the person to grow up. This can cause conflict in the relationship as the child pushes the boundaries and the parents get anxious and overprotective.

Deciding when to share detailed information about the cancer and its follow-up care is an individual decision to be made in each family, but experts agree that by young adulthood, the cancer survivor should know about their disease and follow-up care in order to take on the responsibility of self-care, perhaps in collaboration with the parents or perhaps alone.

———

Sue found herself thinking about The Plan and her experience with cancer a lot over the next few weeks. At nursing school they were still studying the unit on cancer, and she found it a little scary at times. They were learning about the nursing care of people with cancer, and that included children with cancer as well as adults. Some of the reading she did in preparation for class made her feel really sad. She had been one of those children, even though she was fifteen, and reading about the challenges for the family made her realize how much pain her parents had gone through. The other thing that bothered her was thinking about the children who didn't make it. She remembered a boy who had been in the hospital at the same time she was, and how one morning his bed was empty, and the nurses had avoided her questions when she asked about him.

She knew that Dr. Grant was watching her carefully during class, and she tried to keep her emotions in check. She still didn't know what to do about her clinical rotation despite thinking about it over and over. About two days before she was to start her clinical work on the unit, Dr. Grant asked her to stay after class.

"Sue, I'm not sure if you've decided what you want to do about clinical."

"I've been thinking about it, and I don't really know what to do," she replied.

"Well, I talked to some of the other faculty, and what we usually do in these kinds of circumstances is look for an opportunity that is quite different from what you went through. Some suggestions they made include doing a stint in the palliative care unit, although that's not for everyone, or else placing you in an outpatient cancer center. What do you think?"

"I'm not sure I want to go to the cancer center. I still go there for my follow-up care, and I just don't think it would work. I need to think about palliative care some more. I was thinking that being in the children's unit might actually be the best place for me. I was fifteen when I was there, and I don't remember much of it. I was hoping that if I went there, I could maybe work some stuff out for myself."

"Hmm, I have to think about this a bit more." Dr. Grant's face was creased with concern. "This really shouldn't be about you and working stuff out for yourself. You're there to learn and contribute to the work of the unit. Let me think about it, and we can talk some more after class tomorrow, okay?"

Sue nodded. She really was confused about what to do. She understood what Dr. Grant had said about working out her own issues, but she really didn't want to go to the palliative care ward or the cancer center. She supposed she could go to the adult inpatient unit, but she really, really wanted to work with the kids.

Later that day, she received an e-mail from Dr. Grant. They were going to make a special arrangement for her and allow her to work on the pediatric unit. But she had to commit to writing a daily journal about her experience, and she had to meet with the clinical supervisor from the nursing school twice a week to talk about her feelings. She would be spending six weeks doing this clinical rotation, working six hours a day with patients and then another two hours in a postshift conference with the other students. And on top of that, she had to write her journal. It was a lot of work, and she knew that sorting out her feelings might be difficult. But it felt like it was time to do this, and she was pleased that the nursing school was allowing her to do it.

Sue is in a unique position as a childhood cancer survivor. By learning more about her disease and its treatment, she is exposed to both positive and potentially negative opportunities. On the one hand, knowledge is helpful, and what she learns in the classroom may help her understand her cancer experience. On the other hand, it can raise all sorts of anxieties for her too. Anyone who has gone through a significant health challenge should be educated about it, but as a student nurse, Sue is learning far more than the average survivor.

Sue was very nervous the first day of her clinical experience. She barely slept the night before and had to drink two cups of coffee on the way to the hospital to feel awake. She had put out her uniform the night before, but she left her lunch behind in the refrigerator. She could feel her heart beating very fast as she waited for the rest of her clinical group to arrive for their first day. The clinical supervisor was already there, and they used the time while they were waiting to go over what Sue was expected to do in her journal. Jackie—that was the name of the supervisor—explained that all the students would be writing a journal, but Sue was expected to reflect on her feelings as they related to being a patient there seven years ago.

"Sue, if you feel comfortable sharing your experience about when you were here as a patient with the rest of your clinical group, that's fine. They can learn a lot from you. But you don't have to do that. No one need know about your history; that's personal. But if you want to share, that's okay, too. And if you find yourself having any difficulty at all, you must tell me. Is that clear?"

Sue let out a long breath. She hadn't realized that she had been holding her breath while Jackie was talking. "Yes, perfectly clear. Thanks, Jackie. This whole thing means a lot to me, and honestly, I don't know how I'm going to feel. I understand that it's important to keep you in the loop about how it's going for me, and I will."

The first week went by very fast. Sue and the rest of her group spent most of their time shadowing the nurses who worked on the unit. There was a lot to learn, and they were all grateful that they had the chance to observe before they actually had to do anything. They were encouraged to spend time with the young patients, talking and getting to know them. Sue found herself really enjoying this time, but she also noticed that she tended to pick out the younger patients to talk to, not the teenagers. She wrote about this in her journal, and Jackie talked to her about it in private.

"I guess I'm a little nervous to talk to the teenagers. I'm just not sure what it will bring up."

"That's okay, Sue. Just take your time and see how you feel. Tell me about what you've learned so far."

"Well, one thing I've noticed is that the nurses and doctors really involve the kids' parents in decision making about treatment. I was not aware of that when I was in the hospital. Maybe I was just out of things because of the chemo and everything, but maybe my parents kept that away from me. I'm not sure."

"That would be an interesting topic for your final paper, Sue. Have you given that any thought?"

"Not really. I was thinking about doing something about survivorship care plans. Do you know about those? They gave me one, well, actually my parents, when I was discharged from here. My mom has followed it to the letter, and I thought it would be interesting to do my project on that."

"That is interesting. Of course I know about them, but perhaps you could look into the research about them, on a more detailed level."

The Institute of Medicine (IOM) published a report in 2005 titled "From Cancer Patient to Cancer Survivor: Lost in Transition," which has become the definitive guide for survivorship care in North America. This landmark report recognizes survivorship as a distinct phase of the cancer journey, and one that needs to be recognized as such by cancer specialists and other health care providers. A key aspect of providing care for cancer survivors is ensuring that all members of the patient's care team, including the patient and family, know what is expected after primary treatment ends. Knowing what has been done, what needs to be done in the future, and by whom is found to be as important as the details of the recommended plan. The report recommends that every cancer patient be provided with a written survivorship care plan that includes the following components:

1. *A treatment summary with details of the diagnosis, including type of cancer and extent of disease, and a list of the primary treatment provided.*
2. *An ongoing care plan including information about the likely course of recovery, possible short- and long-term effects from the treatments provided, and signs of possible recurrence and second tumors.*
3. *Guidelines for recognizing recurrence or the development of new cancers, which should be based on clinical guidelines where possible.*
4. *A description of long-term effects of treatment so that the patient understands what might happen and will be alert to complications far into the future.*
5. *Non-cancer health care needs should also be addressed. These include recommendations about diet and exercise, alcohol intake, smoking, and immunizations. Cancer survivors increasingly go on to lead full lives, and their health care needs are not limited to those related to the distant cancer.*

6. *Psychosocial concerns are important for quality of life, especially as these may be ignored in light of the urgency of treatment. Psychosocial concerns include depression and anxiety, back-to-work issues, sexuality, family stress and coping, and social isolation.*

7. *Employment, insurance, and economic issues may also be addressed in the survivorship care plan.*

8. *The final part of the care plan, although not necessarily presented last in a written document, is the identification and provision of contact information for all health care providers involved in the patient's care. This is extremely important as it allows the patient to contact specific health care providers if they encounter difficulties or need more information, and it prevents the patient from falling through the cracks when provision of services is not well coordinated.*

The survivorship care plan should be an adaptable tool that can be changed as the patient's needs and circumstances change. For example, for a young woman like Sue, additions can be made at a time when she is considering having a baby. There may be a need for additional testing or surveillance while she is pregnant or if she wants to conceive.

Over the next weeks, Sue spent many hours in the hospital library reading all she could about survivorship care plans. She was surprised to discover that not all cancer patients were given these, and she felt so grateful that she and her parents had one. She made a copy of her own care plan and compared and contrasted the information in it with the recommendations offered by the IOM report. She decided that was what she was going to write her final project about—how her personal care plan compared to the recommendations of the IOM report.

Once she got started on the project, it was interesting and challenging. It felt a little strange to be using her own health information for a school project, but she was not upset by anything she saw in her own care plan. It almost gave her a little distance from her own experience. And she was pleased to see that her care plan met the standards set by the IOM. It was all there—her diagnosis and treatment plan, the tests she had to have in follow-up, recommendations for ongoing surveillance for recurrence and late effects, and the list of health care providers, just as the IOM suggested.

The one area where she felt the information could have been better was psychosocial concerns. There were notes about family stress, but nothing about sexuality or social coping. She thought about that for a while. She was seventeen when her treatment ended, and she guessed that whoever filled out her care plan had assumed that sex was not part of her life. And it wasn't even at twenty-two! She wondered if she should write about that in her project, and then she decided that not only was she going to write about it, but she was going to talk to someone about it during her next follow-up appointment, too.

Sitting at the kitchen table in her home, she felt for the first time that she was ready to be in charge of her own health. Her mother had been in control for so long, but she was really ready now to take over that control. She smiled as she sat there, her laptop open on the table in front of her. She had wanted to be a nurse to help others as she had been helped when she was sick. But she hadn't expected that her studies would ultimately help *her*. She reached out her fingers and started typing again. This was an insight that she just had to put down in her next journal entry.

· 9 ·

We Want to Start a Family

$\mathcal{M}$any cancer survivors have not started or completed childbearing when the cancer diagnosis is made. This can present some significant challenges. David and Lesley are one such couple. When Lesley was diagnosed with non-Hodgkin's lymphoma at age twenty-five, their only thought was to save her life. Now that she is well again, they want to have a baby.

Lesley's diagnosis was confirmed two weeks before her wedding to David. They went ahead with the wedding anyway. She hardly remembers most of it, and when she looks at her wedding pictures, she can see the strain behind her forced smile. David looked like a deer caught in headlights, and her parents could barely smile for the photographer. They didn't tell anyone other than her sister about her cancer until after the wedding. Lesley had to tell her because she was her maid of honor and the person closest to her, other than David, in the whole wide world. They canceled their honeymoon, and instead of going to Hawaii, Lesley spent the next six months having chemotherapy and visiting oncologists. She went into remission after the chemotherapy, and everyone celebrated—everyone except her. She was too weak and sick to celebrate.

Now, two years later, that time is a memory, a painful and stressful memory, but thankfully it is in the past. She applied for a job as a nursery school teacher soon after her treatment was over, and she loves going to work every day. The three- and four-year-old children are so cute, and she loves how they call her "Lelly." David has a great job as a graphic designer for a busy advertising agency. On paper, everything looked perfect. But there was one cloud that hung over their lives. Lesley had been trying for six months to get pregnant, but so far they had not had any success. She had always wanted

131

to have a family, and in her plans, she was going to have two children, a boy and a girl, and she wanted to have them both before she turned thirty. She heard her biological clock ticking loudly. David tried to get her to relax about it, but she just couldn't. She thought about it all the time. Last week, one of the mothers of her nursery school children came to pick up her daughter from school, and Lesley noticed a bump under her sweater. In a flash, she felt the tears rush to her eyes, and she had to turn away and concentrate on something else before she embarrassed herself. In her head she knew that six months wasn't really a long time in the big scheme of things. Some of her friends had tried to get pregnant for much longer. But she was used to getting her way, and she was really trying. She had changed her diet and was now almost a vegetarian. She had read somewhere that this could help her conceive. She told David that he should also cut out meat, and his response was a glare. She didn't want to talk to her mom or sister about it, but she longed for someone to be sympathetic about her situation.

For some women (and men), the drive to have children is so strong that it defies reason. It can be particularly difficult for people who are usually successful, who are driven, and who are used to things going their way. There can often be a big difference between the attitudes of the woman and the man, with the latter feeling less strongly about conceiving and having a baby. This can lead to conflict in the relationship.

She made an appointment to see her family physician. She didn't tell David about it because they often ended up arguing about what he called her "fixation" with getting pregnant. She had known Dr. Harms since she was a teenager, and she really liked her. Even though she had not seen Dr. Harms she was having treatment for her lymphoma, the doctor had called her at home to offer her support. She was a woman in her late fifties, about Lesley's mother's age, and she had a warm smile and a quiet manner. She somehow made Lesley feel safe, and that's what she needed now. She wanted someone to listen to her and make her feel like everything was going to be okay.

Dr. Harms was running late. Lesley had been sitting in the waiting room for almost an hour before she was called in to one of the examination rooms. Dr. Harms rushed into the room, her face flushed and her hair falling out of the ponytail she always wore. She still delivered babies and, as she explained to Lesley, had been up half the night and into the morning with a new baby who was taking his time coming into the world. She was very surprised when Lesley burst into tears.

"What's going on, Lesley?"

"Why can everyone have a baby except *me*?" Her voice rose at the end of her plaintive question. "We've tried and tried, and nothing seems to be working."

"Lesley, just take a deep breath and start from the beginning."

Dr. Harms' calm voice brought Lesley back into the present, and she stopped crying. "Well, we've been trying for six months to get pregnant, and it's not working. I wanted to have my family before I turned thirty, and I'm twenty-seven now. I need to get started on this, but nothing seems to work! Every month it's the same—my damn period shows up like clockwork, and I'm not pregnant! David keeps telling me to relax, but he doesn't understand." Her voice started to go up again, and the tears fell down her face.

"Listen to me carefully, Lesley. What did they tell you when you started treatment for the lymphoma? Did anyone talk to you about fertility after treatment?"

Lesley looked at the doctor with a blank stare. "I don't think so. At least I can't remember. It was such a blur—with the wedding and all. I just remember them talking to me about the kind of chemotherapy I was going to have, and then I started the day after the wedding. Maybe they did, and I didn't take it in. I honestly can't remember."

———

It is not unusual for the time around diagnosis and the beginning of treatment to be a blur. First, being diagnosed with cancer is a huge shock, and then you are often given large amounts of complex information and asked to make a decision about treatment. There are new words and ideas to learn about, and you have to do this when your mind is reeling and your world has been turned upside down.

We know from research that after you have heard the words, "You have cancer," most people are able to take in only 10 percent of what they are told next. No wonder Lesley can't remember if anyone talked to her about the impact of chemotherapy on future childbearing!

———

"Well, we can sort that out with them. You still see the oncologist, right? When is your next appointment?"

"Next week, I think. Maybe I should ask my parents. They came with me to most of the appointments before I started chemo."

"Would David remember?"

Lesley's face crumpled. "I don't really want to ask him. He gets so upset with me when I talk about getting pregnant."

Dr. Harms sat for a moment before answering. It was so ironic that couples who really wanted a baby sometimes struggled, while teenagers seemed to get pregnant at the drop of a hat.

"I understand how upsetting this is for you, Lesley. But this is not *your* problem. David is your husband, and he must be a part of this. It takes two."

"I know. But I don't think he cares about this as much as I do."

"I'm sure he cares a lot about this, and he's probably feeling helpless as well. But I can't speak for him. You need to talk about this together. If I can help you have the conversation together, I am more than willing to be the mediator or facilitator. But in the meantime, I think it would be wise for the two of you to find out from the oncologist if your treatment could play a part. Or it may just be too early—six months really isn't a long time to be trying."

"I don't want to hear that! I'm sorry, Dr. Harms, but six months has been a very long time for me! I want to have a baby *now*, and I don't want to hear about patience or relaxation or giving it time!"

As frustrating as it may be to not conceive exactly when you want to, most doctors will not do anything about the issue until a couple has been trying to conceive for about two years. That can be a very long time when every month brings a woman's period and all she wants is to have skipped it and be pregnant. The doctor is also correct about this being an issue that the couple has to deal with as a couple—it is not just the woman's problem, and she cannot solve it alone.

With that, Lesley ran out of the examination room, through the crowded waiting room, and out into the parking lot. She slammed the car door behind her and sat at the wheel, her breath coming in great gasps. Why did no one understand? She thought about calling the cancer center and bringing her appointment forward, but then she decided that she could wait until next week. It was only five days, really, and she wanted to do a bit of research on her own before she saw the oncologist. As she drove home, she thought about what Dr. Harms had said about David being a part of this, too. She had been thinking of going to her next appointment with the oncologist by herself, but on second thought she decided that David needed to come with her. She would talk to him about it that night.

It was weird, but David seemed almost happy when she asked him to go with her to the oncologist. She didn't tell him that she wanted to ask if the chemotherapy might have affected her ability to conceive, but she was glad that he seemed eager to go with her. The next five days went by quickly. Her work as a nursery school teacher was tiring, but she loved the little kids, and the time at work sped by. Then it was the weekend, and she spent some time on the computer searching for information about fertility after chemotherapy. She was disappointed with most of the information. A lot of it was too general and did not tell her about the effects of the drug combination she had been given. There were a lot of websites for fertility clinics, but she didn't want to think about all that. There were some websites that offered support for couples who could not conceive, and she glanced over them, panic rising in her throat as she read the stories of couples who ended up adopting or spending thousands of dollars on fertility treatments and still not having a baby.

———

One needs to exercise caution when researching any medical topic on the Internet. Although there is a lot of information out there, not all of it is useful or valid. In chapter 12, you will find a list of recommended websites. These are from trusted organizations and associations. But anyone can start a website, and many people do just that, with their personal experience published for all to see. Their opinions are not necessarily reliable or valid and are merely personal expressions. Stories on the Web can be very touching, but they can also be upsetting. Websites that look like legitimate sources of information may be the window dressing of a for-profit agency that wants to hook you in and take your money, with no regard for integrity. If it sounds too good to be true (e.g., "99 percent of our patients conceive in the first month"), then it likely is. Be careful about what you see and assume to be the truth!

———

Lesley still felt sick when she walked into the cancer center. It reminded her of a difficult time in her life, and she actually had a physical reaction to it. As she and David sat down in the waiting room, she felt dizzy, and she broke out in a light sweat. David tried to hold her hand, but it felt clammy and she pulled it away from him.

A short while later, she heard her name being called, and a young woman ushered her into an examination room. The room was quite large, with a desk and two armchairs, an examination table in the far corner, and the usual posters on the walls with advice about exercise and diet. Lesley sat in the chair with her eyes closed, and she tried to control her breathing and heart rate. Both were getting faster by the minute as she waited. It was always like this when she came to the clinic. She would never forget sitting in a room like this when they dropped the bombshell that almost ruined everything. It was here that her world had almost fallen apart when they told her that she had cancer, two weeks before her wedding.

She tried to remind herself that things were different now. She had completed treatment, and she felt better. Her wedding had happened after all. She couldn't feel any enlarged lymph nodes under her arms, and that was a good sign. Up to now, all of her blood work and CT scans had been good. The doctor had told her at her last appointment that she was doing well and that she should stop worrying, or at least not worry so much. As she thought about this, she heard the door open, and before he was even in the room, Dr. Woods was greeting her.

"Lesley, good to see you! Oh, this must be your husband! Nice to meet you after all this time! I was not sure why Lesley didn't bring you to her appointments, but she is one independent young woman!"

Neither Lesley nor David said anything in response. This had been a source of some conflict while Lesley was going through treatment. She had always brought her mom or her sister with her, and in recent months she had come alone. That was the way she wanted it, and David respected her wishes. But he did feel a little bit left out of this experience, and he really wanted to be supportive of her. He didn't have much time to think about that, though, because Lesley had started talking.

"Dr. Woods, what did you tell me about being able to conceive after my treatment?"

The doctor looked at her, his face blank. "I'd have to check in your chart. That's usually done by the nurse."

"I didn't see a nurse! I only saw you once, and then I got married and started chemo! No one told me anything! If I had known, I would have done something else." Her voice was getting shriller with every word, and her face was red. David tried to calm her down by touching her hand, but she pulled away from him. "How could you do this to me? How could you not tell me? This explains everything!"

Dr. Woods raised his hand in the air, almost as if he could physically stop the torrent of pain coming out of her mouth. "Just hang on a minute, young lady! Sit down and take a deep breath! I'm sure we told you the risks of the various agents we were going to use to treat your cancer. Maybe you just didn't hear. There was a lot you had to take in at that first meeting, and it's quite common to forget things. And anyway, the treatment we gave you usually doesn't affect fertility in the long run. So just stop yelling and calm down!"

The impact of chemotherapy on future fertility should be discussed with every patient of childbearing age, and it should also be discussed with the parents of children diagnosed with cancer. But in the crisis of the moment, three things can happen: First, the newly diagnosed person may not want to talk about it. When your life is threatened by cancer, you may not consider future fertility to be as important. For the parents of a young child with cancer, this may be the furthest thing from their minds as they face the potential loss of their precious child. Second, the health care provider may decide that it is not an important topic to be discussed. This is a paternalistic attitude, but it does exist. And third, the discussion may be initiated in a very superficial way or the patient may not be able to take it all in, given the large amount of information to be absorbed in such a short time frame. Any or all of these may be the reason that Lesley can't remember being told about fertility after treatment.

In a nationwide study of oncologists, 30 percent said that they rarely consider a woman patient's desires for fertility when planning treatment. Their focus is on curing the cancer. Less than half of the oncologists in another study routinely referred their female cancer patients to a specialist in fertility preservation. Other studies have found that between one- and two-thirds of women with cancer are not told about the effects of treatment on fertility, and those who are told want even more information than they are given.

———

Lesley was sitting on the edge of the chair. Her eyes were blazing, and her cheeks flushed. David didn't know what to do. He was a little embarrassed that she had yelled at the doctor, and he was also mad that she hadn't told him that she was going to talk about this to the oncologist. He didn't know why she was so worked up about not being pregnant. He was not sure that he was ready for a baby yet, and he also wasn't sure that it would be good for her health to get pregnant so soon after finishing her treatment. And he really thought that this was a private matter that the two of them should sort out, not something that should be broadcast to the world.

Dr. Woods started talking again. "To put your mind at rest, I'm going to refer you to a specialist, a reproductive endocrinologist. They'll explain everything to you and likely do some tests. But I want to repeat myself again—the regimen that you had does not lead to infertility."

Lesley sat back in her chair. At least the doctor was taking her seriously. She hardly listened as he went through the results of her latest blood tests. She sat silently as he felt her neck and under her arms for enlarged lymph nodes. And then he was gone, the door closing with a hiss behind him. She could hardly look at David. She knew his face would have that pinched look it got when he was mad at her. She'd been seeing that pinched look a lot lately.

A couple of days later she received a call from the reproductive endocrinology clinic. They would see her the next week. She was both excited and scared at the prospect. What if the news was bad and she couldn't conceive? She had been visiting some websites on the Internet and had the names and addresses of some fertility clinics in the city where they lived. The websites were very professional looking, and they all had photos and testimonials from satisfied customers. At least she had that to fall back on! She hadn't shown David any of this. He was acting like he was still mad at her, and he came home late most nights. He told her they were working on a big project at work, but she was not sure she believed him.

"Do you want to come with me to see the specialist?" she asked the night before her appointment.

"Do you *want* me to come with you?" was his reply.

They stared at each other for a few seconds. David was usually a calm person, but he felt himself getting angry often these days, and this was one of those times.

"Do whatever you want," Lesley retorted and left the room.

———

Infertility is known to cause significant conflict for many couples. Even though no cause may be found for the infertility, the couple may blame each other. There are also significant costs associated with the diagnosis and treatment of infertility, which can put additional strain on the partnership. As we see with Lesley and David, she is much more interested in having a baby, and he is more ambivalent. This difference in itself can be the source of much unhappiness.

———

The next morning when she got out of the shower, she found David in the kitchen sitting at the table and eating a large bowl of cereal. He usually left the house by 7:30 to avoid the worst of the traffic, so this meant he was planning on coming with her. He looked up from his bowl and greeted her.

"Les, I really don't want us to fight about this. I just feel left out of so many things that are going on in your life. This is *our* life, and I don't want you to be alone in any of this."

"Then why aren't you more supportive of me?" Her voice was getting shrill, and that often meant that she was going to cry.

"I'm trying to be supportive, but most of the time I don't know what's going on in your head. You don't talk to me about what you're thinking. You've never asked me what I want with this baby business."

"It's not 'baby business' David!" I want to have a baby. For us. You should want to have one, too!"

"Well, you've never asked me what I want!"

"I can't get into this now. My appointment is in forty-five minutes, and I need to be calm for this. You're welcome to come with me, but please let's not fight all the way there."

"Well, at least we agree on that."

They drove to the appointment in silence. The specialist's office was on the other side of the downtown area, and traffic was heavy until they left the highway and got onto a feeder road. David drove, and Lesley sat with her hands clenching her purse. Her knuckles were white, and she had a difficult time opening the car door when they pulled into the parking spot outside a tall modern building.

They rode the elevator to the fifth floor in silence. They waited only a short time in the modern waiting room before they were ushered into a well-decorated office. They both looked around at the modern artwork on the walls, but before they could take it all in, a youngish man in a white coat entered the room.

"Hello! I'm Chris Summer. Pleased to meet you. I see that you're a patient of Dr. Woods. He's a good man. Now, why don't you tell me why you're here?"

Lesley hesitated. She already felt the tears beginning to choke her, and she wanted to be in control for this appointment. "Well, I was treated for non-Hodgkin's lymphoma about two years ago, and I want to have a baby. But nothing's happened."

"Hmm. How long have you been trying to conceive?"

"Well, about six months, I guess. Please don't tell me that it's too soon! That's what everyone says. I don't know why they didn't talk to me about this before my chemo. Maybe they could have done something to prevent this from happening!"

"Well, it may be too soon. But before we jump to any conclusions, there are some blood tests that I want you to have that will tell us if your hormone levels are in the normal range. If they aren't, then we can correct them and see if that helps. We'll do this in a stepwise fashion, not skipping any of the steps. There is no evidence that the chemotherapy regimen you were given affects fertility, so this may not be related to that at all. This is going to take some time, so please have patience."

"Dr. Summer, I read about these treatments that a woman can have to help her get pregnant. I read about it here." Lesley dug around in her purse and pulled out a sheaf of paper that she had printed off the Internet. He glanced at them quickly and replied:

"Now Lesley, I told you to have patience. These treatments may be useful for women with established infertility. We don't know that you have that."

"Come on, Les, let's go get the blood tests." David was embarrassed at her open desperation.

"That's a good idea," Dr. Summer said. "We'll set up another appointment for you for early next week where we'll go over the results and see what comes next."

The specialist held the door of the office open for them; the appointment was over.

Dealing with infertility can be very frustrating and is a source of distress for most couples who experience it. Couples faced with infertility have levels of depression twice those of the normal population. Emotional well-being, relationship satisfaction, and sexuality are also compromised.

For women whose fertility may be negatively affected by cancer treatment, deciding what to do can be very difficult. Complex decisions have to be made in a time of crisis. Fertility-preserving options have to be weighed against life-saving treatment. And the options for fertility preservation for women are limited.

The best option for a woman with cancer whose treatment may affect her fertility is to harvest her eggs and create embryos with her partner's sperm. The embryos are then frozen for implantation at a future time. This method is the most successful (with a greater than 50 percent chance of success), but there are draw-backs. Treatment for the cancer has to be delayed for at least one menstrual cycle, and the woman has to take medication to stimulate the ovaries to produce multiple eggs. This is done with hormones, and women with hormone-dependent cancers usually should not be exposed to additional hormones. It is also dependent on having a partner who can donate sperm for fertilization.

There are other strategies for preserving fertility in women, but these remain experimental, with very low levels of success. They include freezing eggs (with a less than 4 percent chance of success) and freezing ovarian tissue that is put back into the woman after treatment is complete (still experimental due to very limited success so far).

For women who need pelvic radiation as treatment, it is common practice to shield the ovaries from the field of radiation or even to move them surgically out of the radiation field. Radiation to the pelvis may result in anatomical changes to the uterus, so even if the woman is able to become pregnant, the chances of a successful outcome are limited by the ability of the uterus itself to hold a pregnancy.

The best option for fertility preservation is for men with cancer. Freezing sperm for later use is a highly successful and well-established practice. However, the man must know about this option before *treatment starts and must have enough time to donate sperm samples (usually two or three times, forty-eight hours apart) and have them frozen. In the rush to begin treatment, this does not always happen, and an op-portunity is lost. For young men and boys, the reality of one day having children just may not be something that they consider important, and so it is not done.*

She went immediately to have the blood drawn, and as she watched the red blood fill the tube, she said a silent prayer. Her visit to the endocrinologist hadn't really given her any answers. Now she had to wait to see if her hormones were normal, and then what? She could see that David wanted to talk about something, but she just blocked him out. He would try to be all reasonable and logical, and this was anything but reasonable and logical for her. She wanted a baby with every cell of her body, and she was determined that she would find a way to have one.

The rest of the week dragged by slowly. She and David hardly talked. He came home late, and she was so exhausted most nights that she went to bed before nine o'clock. It wasn't physical exhaustion; it was emotional. She thought about not being pregnant every moment of the day. And each day her distress increased. One moment, she felt very sad, and the next angry. She thought she might be depressed and wondered what she should do about it. Then she thought that if only she could get pregnant, everything would be fine, and the bad feelings would disappear.

Every morning when she woke up, she lay in bed and took one day off an imaginary calendar in her head. One day less until her appointment with Dr. Summer, one day less before she would have some answers. She imagined what it would be like to be pregnant, to grow a baby inside her. She imagined what the baby would look like, and in her head she put together a composite of her and David's best features. Eventually she would have to stop daydreaming and get up to go to work, and she did so with an aching heart.

———✖———

This longing for children is seen commonly among women diagnosed with cancer. Loss of fertility is often experienced with the same kind of pain as receiving a cancer diagnosis. Women who have had cancer want children for the same reasons as unaffected women—but it is also a way of reclaiming a normal life and a desire to achieve the goals they had before they had cancer.

For women who already have children before their cancer diagnosis, the desire to have more children remains, if that was their plan. The cancer seems to enhance the value of being a parent.

———✖———

Eventually the day of the appointment arrived. David picked her up from work, and they drove to the endocrinology clinic together. He could tell that she was all wound up. She seemed to radiate electricity she was so tense, and so he kept his mouth shut. He was nervous, too, although she didn't seem to realize how this was affecting him. He wasn't sure what he hoped would happen at this appointment. Would it be better if her hormones were normal or if there was something wrong with them? What if there was nothing that could be done? This was not what he imagined marriage would be like. He didn't imagine that cancer would be part of the early days of their marriage, either, but at least with that they knew how long the treatments would last. This quest for a baby was going on longer than the treatment, and from his perspective, it was much more difficult. He felt guilty even thinking these thoughts and made a promise to himself that he would be more supportive of her.

Once again they entered the plush and modern offices of the reproductive endocrinologist. And once again Dr. Summer swept into the room with a sheaf of papers in his hands.

"Good afternoon! I have good news for you. All your tests are normal, completely normal! I'm going to go over them in detail with you, but this is very good news."

David didn't know what to think or feel. He looked over at Lesley, and she didn't look thrilled. Her face was slack, and her eyes had that glazed look she sometimes got when she was pulling away from him. The doctor pointed at numbers on the paper as he spoke, and David tried to appear as if he were concentrating on the words that were swirling around his ears. He could tell that Lesley wasn't paying any attention at all, which was a bit strange. As soon as the doctor stopped talking, Lesley asked one question:

"So there's nothing you can do for me?"

"I see no reason from these results why you shouldn't conceive. It has only been six months, so you should keep trying. If after a year . . ."

Before he could finish his sentence, Lesley got up from her chair and left the room. Dr. Summer seemed startled by her abrupt—and to David, rude—departure.

"I'd best go after her. She gets upset easily. Sorry, sorry."

So David rushed after her. He was not sure how he felt, but he knew that she hadn't received the news she wanted to hear. What did she want to hear? That her hormones were abnormal? How could she want that? She was so hard to predict these days, so different from the carefree and fun person she used to be. He knew that the cancer had knocked the axis of her world off kilter. Of course it had! But it was over, wasn't it?

He found her standing next to the elevator. He reached out his hand to touch her shoulder, but she moved away. They rode down to the main floor in silence, standing on opposite sides of the elevator like strangers. He watched the blinking lights on the panel as the elevator passed down the floors, and then they were out of the building and walking toward the car.

"Just don't say anything, okay, David? Not a damn word! I need to think this through!"

It is not unusual for couples experiencing difficulty in getting pregnant to have significant stress and strain in the relationship. There is sometimes a discordance in the degree to which the members of the couple want to have children, and this can result in conflict and even relationship breakdown. Most fertility clinics have a social worker or psychologist on staff, and a meeting with these professionals is an integral part of the treatment plan. Recognition of the stress that infertility places on a couple is the first step in supporting couples as they enter treatment.

The ride home was silent. Lesley even turned off the radio. David kept looking over at her, but her face was like a stone statue, giving away no clue about what she was thinking or how she was feeling. When they got home, she went into the study, closed the door, and stayed there until he eventually gave up and went to work at 6:30 in the evening. He stayed there until almost midnight, and when he came home she was asleep in their bed.

The next morning she called the nursery school and told them she was coming down with something. As soon as David left for work, she went back to the study and spent an hour on the computer again. She made some phone calls and left the house at ten o'clock precisely. Thirty minutes later she was outside a small building on the edge of the medical campus. The sign over the door said "FAMILY FERTILITY CLINIC." She drew in a deep breath and walked toward the glass doors under the sign.

One hour later she came out, this time with a shiny folder in her hands. She walked to her car and sat there for a few minutes. She glanced at her watch a couple of times and took out her cell phone. Before she dialed, she hesitated, shook her head, and put her cell phone back in her purse. She started the car, backed out of the parking space, and drove home. It was lunchtime, and she was hungry. She made some toast and sat at the kitchen table, absently eating while looking over the materials from the fertility clinic. There was one sheet of paper that she couldn't bring herself to look at again. It was the estimate of costs, and the number on the paper had a lot of zeroes.

She spent the afternoon planning what she was going to say to David. She knew he would be mad that she had gone to the clinic without him. Well, he would be mad that she hadn't even told him that she was going. But she had to do it. She thought about what his response might be and tried to prepare a counterargument to all his objections. Yes, it was a lot of money, but they told her there was a really good chance it would work after the first cycle of drugs. It was a lot of money, but how could you put a dollar value on the life of a child, on their starting a family?

She put a bottle of his favorite white wine in the fridge and made a big salad. Maybe if he had to chew a lot, he wouldn't be able to talk her out of it. She knew she was being silly, but she wanted this really bad. She thought about other times in their life when she had felt really strongly about something and had to persuade him, but there was really nothing. They had agreed about most things over the course of their relationship. But this was different. She knew she could get him to come around, but she was not sure how they were going to find the money.

He had not come home by 6:30. Perhaps he was working late again. She called his cell phone, and he seemed surprised to hear from her.

"David, I made dinner. Are you coming home soon?"

"Um, I was planning to stay here a bit longer. I guess I can come home for dinner and then come back to finish off."

Lesley hesitated. She wanted them to have a good discussion, to sort things out properly, and if he was going to be distracted by what he had left behind, that wouldn't work.

"Could you maybe stay and come home a bit earlier? Like by nine maybe? I want to talk to you about something important."

He felt a sinking feeling in his stomach. She wanted to talk about this baby stuff. Again. He agreed and tried to focus on his work, but it wasn't possible with the threat of a "big talk" hanging over him. So by eight he packed up what he was doing and drove home. Lesley had put linen napkins on the table, and she had a bottle of wine in the fridge. She seemed a little startled to see him home an hour early, and she fussed in the kitchen for a few minutes, tossing the salad and putting some bread in the oven to warm.

As soon as he put the first forkful of salad in his mouth, she began:

"David, I don't want you to get mad. Well, I won't blame you if you do. Just sit there and listen, okay? I went to a fertility clinic today. Please, don't say anything! Just let me tell you what happened, and then you can say what you want. So, I went to see them, and they had great news. I told them about the results from Dr. Summer, and they said that my cancer should not have anything to do with getting pregnant. They showed me their stats, and they have a really good success rate. They said it would probably only take one cycle. They said they would first try with artificial insemination using your sperm, and if that didn't work, then they would do something called IVF—mixing your sperm and my eggs—and then we would have embryos that would be frozen that we could use to have more babies! Isn't that great?"

David sat silently, his jaw moving as he tried to calm himself. You bet he was angry! He was so angry that he could barely think. He managed to get just three words out of his clenched teeth.

"How much, Lesley?"

"It's always about the money with you, isn't it? Why can't you see the big picture? This is about our family!"

"Just answer me, please!"

"Well, it depends on what they do. But if we have to have the IVF, and only if, it's about $15,000." Her voice was very soft as she pronounced the figure.

"Fifteen? Thousand? You're kidding me, right? We don't have that kind of money!"

"They said that they work out a financing plan so we don't have to pay it all up front. Just a deposit and then monthly payments."

"I can't talk right now, Lesley. First you just go off to this clinic on your own without even talking to me. And then you drop this on me like a bomb! I'm not sure that I even know you anymore. What happened to us? We used to talk about everything, and now you do this without telling me that you're even thinking about it!"

"You knew I was thinking about it! You're just in denial! You don't listen to a word I say about the baby. If I start to talk about it, you just shut down. Yes, you came to see the doctor with me last week, but you weren't really there. You were totally checked out!"

"Les, just think about it! Fifteen grand! And that's probably just for one try. And no one has said to you that you can't get pregnant naturally! I guess it would help if we made love occasionally! When was the last time, Les? You've been so damned obsessed with getting pregnant that you forgot what you need to do to get pregnant!"

He pushed his chair away from the table and stormed out of the house. It was a small house, and the walls shook as the door slammed behind him. Lesley stood where she was, tears fighting with her anger to come to the surface. How dare he? After all she had been through! She just wanted to scream, she was so angry! She picked up his plate from the table and threw it across the kitchen. It shattered against the cupboard door, and vegetables glistening with oil flew all over. She sat down where David had been sitting, put her head in her hands, and howled.

After she cried till she had no more tears, she cleaned up the kitchen and went to bed. David didn't come home that night. She knew he was at work, and they had some couches there for people when they pulled all-nighters. In the morning she showered and went to work as usual. During her break she called Dr. Harms' office. The receptionist must have heard something in her voice and offered her the last appointment of the day for that afternoon. Lesley was not sure what she was going to say to her family doctor. She didn't have much time to plan, but she wanted someone who could be objective to give her guidance.

———

What has happened here is not uncommon. Lesley and David are not communicating effectively and instead end up fighting. This is a couples' issue and should be dealt with as a couple. One person trying to get their own way is not an effective solution. Their fighting is also reflective of David's ambivalence and Lesley's strong drive to start a family.

The fertility clinic where Lesley went was also not completely honest with her. They presented (or she heard) very optimistic statistics about the success of assisted reproduction. They made her promises that may not be fulfilled. Care should be taken when choosing a fertility clinic or doctor. It really is "buyer beware" because not all clinics are run by credible doctors. Treating infertility is a business for some, and people desperate to have children can be cheated by false promises and statistics.

It is important to check the credentials of the doctors at any clinic by seeing if they are associated with the American Society of Reproductive Medicine (www .asrm.org) or with an academic teaching hospital. This will in part help to ensure that the doctors associated with the clinic are well qualified.

———◆◇◆———

The day went by quickly, and Lesley was soon on her way to Dr. Harms' office. The waiting room was almost empty when she got there, and she only had to wait ten minutes before being shown into an examination room. Dr. Harms looked flustered as usual, and she sat down in the chair with a big sigh.

"Whew, it's nice to sit down for a minute. How are you, Lesley? David not with you today?"

It was exactly the wrong thing to say, although she couldn't possibly know that. Lesley burst into tears. Between her gasps and sobs, she told Dr. Harms about the events of the past few weeks. The doctor listened and didn't interrupt until Lesley stopped to take a shuddering breath.

"Lesley, I know from the last time you were here that you are upset about this. And what I am going to tell you may not be what you want to hear. But I want you to listen to me, really listen. I have the report from Dr. Woods with the results of your blood work. As I'm sure he told you, everything is normal. That is good news. I understand that you are desperate to have a baby. I really do. But you have to give it a chance. Six months is not a long time to be trying to conceive. Any reproductive specialist worth his or her salt would say the same thing. If you have not conceived after one year of trying—and I mean really trying—then an investigation of the cause is warranted. You've told me that your periods are regular, and your hormone levels are fine. Tell me something, are you and David having sex regularly? This may sound like a stupid question, but . . ."

Lesley looked at her hands. The truth was that they had not made love in a really long time. She had been so mad at him these past weeks that they hadn't even slept in the same bed most of the time. She tried to recall if they'd had sex since her last period, and she couldn't recall if they had.

"Maybe not so regularly. We've been fighting a lot. And he's been working on a big project."

"That may be the first thing you need to do. Make up with your husband, and make love more than just occasionally. Now, the worst thing you could do is make sex something you have to do, like washing the windows! And it can be difficult when you are trying to conceive. But you have to give it a good shot. You are both young and healthy, and there is every reason to believe that it will happen with time. Now is not the time to be going to fertility clinics."

—∞∞∞—

Many couples find that in the effort to conceive, sex becomes mechanical and a chore. Men may experience difficulties getting erections because of the pressure to perform. What used to be fun and an expression of mutual love becomes an exercise that has to be performed even when the desire is not there. This can have long-lasting effects on the relationship, and it can be a challenge to maintain a healthy balance between making love and making a baby.

—∞∞∞—

"But the fertility clinic gives us our best shot!"

"Lesley—listen to me. If, and it's a big if, you need a fertility clinic, then I would refer you to Dr. Summer's clinic. They have an excellent reputation and are associated with the medical school. I trust them, and they are on the cutting edge of fertility treatments. But it is too early for that. What you need to do now is to go home and talk to David. Really talk to him. The two of you sound as if you are on different planets."

"You're right about that. It's as if I hardly know him anymore. And he said the same thing about me last night. Dr. Harms, how did this happen to us?"

"Things happen when couples stop talking. When I was much younger and we didn't have the techniques to help women conceive that we do now, one of my mentors used to tell women with infertility to stop trying so hard. She used to tell them to take a vacation and then get a puppy. The vacation helped them to relax, and they had sex. And the puppy seemed to bring out their mothering instincts, and maybe even helped their hormones—completely unscientific of course! You'd be surprised how many women that worked for."

"David's allergic to dogs, so that's out of the question, even if I thought it would work. And there's no way we could take a vacation. David says we don't have the money for the fertility clinic, so I guess I just have to wait it out. Do you promise to send me back to Dr. Summers if I'm not pregnant in a year?"

"Yes, I promise. Now go home and talk to that husband of yours. And start with an apology."

Lesley glared at the doctor, but then she smiled, just a small smile that caught the corners of her mouth. Perhaps he had been acting out a little, and she really hated it when she and David fought. She thanked Dr. Harms and left the office. On her way home she stopped at the grocery store and bought some food for dinner. It took her a while to plan what she was going to make—perhaps some nice fish, which was a favorite of David's. And she would bake some potatoes and maybe have some green beans. She did not want to make a salad. The memory of the lettuce and tomatoes flying around the kitchen last night was still too fresh.

When she got home, it was close to six o'clock, and she was surprised to see David's car in the driveway. She'd tried calling him from her car, but he didn't pick up. He'd come home early all by himself! Lesley sat in the car for a moment, trying to figure out how to apologize to him for her behavior. She wasn't going to apologize for wanting a baby so badly, just for being so crazy about it. The lights were on in the house, and the first thing she saw was his duffel bag standing in the center of the entrance hall.

"David?" she called as she put down the grocery bags. "Where are you? Why's your bag here?"

There was silence. She walked into the kitchen. He was not there. She looked into the living room, but that was empty too. She thought she heard something from the back of the house, and she walked quickly toward the bedroom. He was in the study, sitting in the chair at the desk, with his back to the hallway. He was writing something by hand, his back curved over the desktop in concentration.

"What are you doing?" she asked, her voice louder than she wanted it to be.

He swiveled around in the chair, his face blank except for the lines that were etched deeply around his mouth. He was only thirty-five, but tonight he looked older and sadder.

"I was just leaving you a note. I didn't know where you were. Les, I think we need a break. I just can't do this anymore. The fighting and the silences are just too much for me. I'm sorry. You've been through a lot, but this is just too much for me. I think you know it, too."

"David, no! For goodness' sake! Don't do this! I'm sorry, I really am. I've been a giant bitch. I bought some fish for dinner. And potatoes. Please, can we just eat and talk about it?"

"I'm not sure there's anything else to say. You talk and talk, and I just don't understand what you're saying. Well, I do understand that you want a baby, but at what cost, Les? And I'm not just talking about the money for the fertility clinic. I feel cut out of all of this. This is about what *you* want! Always *you*. I'm nowhere in this, Les. I just can't do it anymore!"

"But listen, David! I went to Dr. Harms today."

"See? You've done it again. You've gone off to see the doctor, and I didn't even know you were going! Maybe I wanted to go with you! Maybe I wanted to be a part of whatever it is that you were going to talk to her about. But did you ask me to go with you? Did you even think about *me* in this?"

"But David—she told me that I had to apologize. She told me that . . ."

"So you're apologizing because she told you to? It's not even you doing something because you realized you were wrong? This is just another example of what's wrong between us, Les!"

"That came out all wrong, David. What I meant to say is that she told me some things that helped me realize . . ."

"Not now, Les. I just can't hear it now. I'm going to leave now. I packed a bag. I'm going to stay at my brother's for a while. I'll call you next week, and maybe then we can try and talk. I have to do this, for myself this time. I just can't go on like this, Les. I just can't."

He got up from the chair, his unfinished note shining bright white under the lamp. Lesley remained where she was, her feet stuck to the floor as if they were magnetized. She didn't hear the door close behind him, but the sounds of his footsteps echoed in the empty house for a long time. She was more alone than she had ever been in her whole life. And it felt terrible.

· *10* ·

Am I Losing My Mind?

$\mathcal{A}$fter the months of treatment when life is anything but normal, many cancer survivors want to pick up the pieces and be like they were before. For those who have had chemotherapy, some cognitive changes may result, and these can interfere with memory, language, and other activities involving the brain. Cancer-related cognitive changes (sometimes called chemo-brain) are one of the challenges of life after cancer.

Gail is fifty-two years old and a two-year survivor of breast cancer. She is also a nurse with thirty years of experience. She works in a busy medical ward at a teaching hospital and is very proud of her relationships with her patients and with her colleagues. When she was diagnosed with breast cancer, she was really shocked. She somehow always thought that taking care of patients would protect her. The months of diagnosis and treatment were a blur. She had a lumpectomy and then radiation followed by nine months of chemotherapy. She took almost a year off work, and for the past fourteen months has been back on the ward—thinner and fatigued, but back.

It hasn't been easy for her. Working full time is physically and mentally exhausting, but the year off took a chunk out of her savings. Retirement is looking like a distant mirage. Her husband, Jim, is a teacher, and they have only a small nest egg put away. She has to work, but there are limited opportunities for part-time positions at the hospital. So she just has to bite the bullet. Most days she comes home from her shift and collapses in a chair, unable to even think about making dinner. Jim is really easygoing, so he often warms up some soup and makes toast, and that's what they have for dinner.

Gail expected that it would take a while to get back to her old self. Everyone told her that this was how it would be, and at first she believed them. The physical exhaustion has gotten better, but she is still not sleeping well.

151

Soon after the chemotherapy was over, her oncologist put her on antiestrogen medication, and she has to take this for five years. The chemotherapy put her into menopause, and the medication has made the hot flashes worse. She wakes up three or four times a night, drenched in sweat, and then shivers as she tries to find a dry spot on the bed to fall asleep on. She wakes in the morning to the insistent buzzing of the alarm and can barely get up to get ready. Once she's showered and has had some coffee on the way to work, she feels more awake, but the nights of broken sleep are taking their toll.

Every Monday morning on her unit, there is a team meeting where the nurses and doctors sit down together and review the patients who were admitted over the weekend. They also discuss the other patients and review their treatment plans and progress. Gail finds it difficult to concentrate in these meetings. Her mind wanders, and she has to try very hard to focus on what is being said. Last week she sat through the whole meeting and hardly heard a word. At one point, Dr. Henderson asked her a question about a patient, and she had to ask him to repeat himself. She was very embarrassed and struggled for a few moments to answer. Then Julie, one of her colleagues, covered for her.

"Gail was probably not involved in that patient's admission, Dr. Henderson. I think Penny was, but she's off today. Let me look in the patient's chart for that information."

Gail breathed a big sigh of relief. Dr. Henderson had once yelled at a nurse in one of these meetings, and she didn't want to be the next person who got yelled at. He had a short temper and was often rude to the nurses, but zoning out during the meeting was no excuse. She thanked Julie afterward.

"I'm not sure where my head was when Dr. H. asked me about that patient. Thanks for covering for me. I owe you one."

Julie smiled and patted Gail on the shoulder. This was not the first time that Gail had been unfocused in a team meeting, and Julie didn't know what to say. They were all friends on the unit, and a core group of them had worked together for more than eight years. Other nurses came and went, but there were three of them who had started almost at the same time: Gail, Julie, and Susan. It was difficult for all of them when Gail was first diagnosed with breast cancer. They were like sisters, and her pain affected them all. They supported her when she went through treatment and were happy when she returned to work. But Julie was worried that everything was not as it should be with her friend, and she decided to talk to Susan about it. They took their lunch break together that day, and Julie suggested they go outside to eat their sandwiches.

"This is strange," Susan commented as they left the building and walked into the bright sunshine. "You usually hate leaving the unit. What's up?"

"I wanted to talk to you about Gail. Something happened this morning at the team meeting, and I'm worried about her. Have you noticed anything different about her?"

Susan sighed. She didn't say anything for a moment as they sat down on a bench. "She's definitely not herself, that's for sure. I wondered if you had noticed, but I just didn't say anything. What have you seen?"

"Well, this morning it was as if she was totally zoned out. Dr. H. asked her about a patient, and she didn't have a clue what he was talking about. I covered for her, but this is not the first time something like this has happened."

"I know. I've seen it, too. Maybe she has chemo-brain. You know, like my mom had after her cancer. She had difficulty remembering stuff, and she had zero concentration. Maybe Gail has that, too."

The two of them sat in silence for a while, their sandwiches lying untouched in their laps. Perhaps Gail had been affected by her treatment. The thought worried them both.

Chemo-brain is more accurately known as "cancer- or cancer-treatment-associated cognitive change." Changes in cognition can occur at any point in the cancer journey. For some, the crisis of diagnosis causes an inability to concentrate as well as forgetfulness. Radiation or surgery to the brain itself may lead to cognitive changes as a result of direct damage to the brain. Chemotherapy can also impact brain functioning, though the mechanism for this is not yet clearly described. What is known, however, is that many people report changes in their cognitive functioning as a result of treatment for cancer.

"So what are we going to do about this?" Susan was always the one who looked for immediate action on things. It was one of her strengths, and Julie was relieved when she asked the question.

"I think we should talk to Gail before we do anything else. After that, we should maybe talk to Rosemary. She's the manager, and she may have seen something, too. Or maybe others have said something to her about Gail. Oh, this is just awful!"

Neither of them had eaten their lunch, and they slowly wrapped their sandwiches, put them back in their lunch bags, and walked back toward the doors of the hospital. When they got back to their unit, Gail was standing at the nurses' station, a pen in her hand and a patient's chart in front of her. She seemed deep in thought, so the two women walked past her and into the lunchroom. As they left after putting their lunch bags into the refrigerator, Gail stopped them.

"Where did you two go? I waited for you for lunch, but I couldn't find you. Did you eat? I didn't because I wanted to have lunch with you, and now there's a new admission."

"Um, we thought we'd eat outside, but it was too hot. So we haven't eaten either. Can I help you with the admission and then maybe we can eat a bit later? I'm starving."

Julie felt bad that she and Susan had left their friend behind. They usually ate their lunches together, a hurried fifteen-minute break from the busy unit and their duties.

"That would be great! I could use some help with this new patient. She's eighty-five years old and really confused. She keeps wandering out of her room, and I haven't been able to get a sensible word out of her. I think her daughter is on her way, and she might be able to give me a history on her. Could you do her blood pressure and get her into bed while I wait for her daughter?"

Julie nodded and walked quickly down the hallway to find the new patient. She found a rather agitated elderly lady in the room and with her was another woman who looked to be about sixty years old.

"Hello, I'm Julie, one of the nurses on this unit. I'm here to help you get comfortable. Can you tell me your name?"

The older woman didn't reply, but an answer came from the person who was with her. "Hello, Julie. I'm Beth, and this is my mom, Lilly Morgan. Mom, do you want to say hello to the nurse? Her name's Julie, just like your great-granddaughter."

As Julie waited for the patient to answer, she was sure that Gail had said the patient's daughter had not arrived yet. How strange. Well, perhaps Gail had not seen her come into the unit. The elderly lady seemed not to have heard the question and was standing next to the bed, her bony fingers stroking the crisp white sheets.

"I don't think it's her hearing," the daughter said. "But she hardly responds to us anymore. She ignores me, like she did just now. It's getting more and more difficult."

"I expect it must be. Why is she being admitted today?"

Just before the daughter could answer, Gail entered the room. She appeared flustered, and her hands were empty. "Did I leave the chart in here? Has anyone seen it?"

Julie shook her head. "I saw you with it at the desk. Did you take it away from there?"

"No, I just can't find it. I had it a few minutes ago, and then I turned around and it was gone. Damn it, this is irritating. I wish people would just leave things alone!"

She walked quickly out of the room, leaving Julie and the patient's daughter staring at her back.

"If you'll excuse me a moment, I'm going to help Gail find that chart. Gail will be looking after your mother for the rest of the day. I'm just helping her. I'll see you in a few minutes."

Julie stood outside the patient's room and watched as Gail searched the desk at the nurses' station. Even down the hallway, she could see the chart sitting on top of the raised portion of the desk, but somehow Gail could not see where she had left it. She walked toward the desk. She could see that Gail was getting more frustrated by the second. She picked up the chart and offered it to her friend.

"Is this what you're looking for?"

"Where did you find it? Are you playing tricks on me?"

"Uh, no. It was here, on top of the desk. You were writing in it a while ago."

"Well, someone must have moved it when I wasn't looking and then put it back. This is so irritating! Why do people touch things that don't have anything to do with them?"

Julie said nothing, but a sick feeling crept into her stomach. Why and how had Gail missed that? The chart had been there all along, and she had not seen it. This was unusual for Gail who had always been on top of everything. It was really not like her.

Cancer-related cognitive changes can present themselves in different ways. Some people may have difficulty concentrating, staying focused, or paying attention. Gail's inability to focus and concentrate while sitting in a meeting is typical of this problem. Visual memory can also be affected, and a perfect example of this is the situation where Gail forgets where she put the patient's chart. These signs can be quite subtle and may be attributed to other causes, such as poor sleep, fatigue, or just making a mistake. However, when there is a pattern or these signs are consistent, it is likely due to something other than coincidence.

Julie continued with her own work for the rest of the day. She kept an eye out for her friend, but Gail seemed to spend most of the afternoon in the patients' rooms and did not ask for help again. Eventually the end of shift came, and the three nurses, Gail, Julie, and Susan, walked out of the hospital and to their cars together. Gail was pale and looked exhausted. She hardly spoke as they walked and the other two chatted about their day.

"Is something wrong?" Susan asked.

"I'm just wiped out by the end of the shift," Gail replied. "These twelve-hour shifts really take it out of me."

"They are brutal," Julie agreed. "I sometimes wonder how you manage, after the treatment and everything."

"I just wish I could get a decent night's sleep. The damned hot flashes are a real problem. I can't remember the last time I had a full night's sleep."

As she talked, Julie felt her concerns about her colleague lessen. It must be the lack of sleep that makes her forgetful, she thought, nothing else.

———

Poor-quality sleep or sleep that is disturbed can play a role in one's ability to cope and be efficient during the day. Hot flashes at night are sometimes called night sweats because they cause excessive sweating that wakes the person up. They are often associated with menopause and can be particularly bad for women who have been put into menopause by chemotherapy. They are also often very bad for women who take antiestrogen medication as part of their treatment for breast cancer. A lack of estrogen in a woman's body is known to cause hot flashes and can be extremely bothersome.

———

The next day at work, Gail looked even more tired. Her skin was pale, and she had dark circles under her eyes. Julie was busy most of the day with an unstable patient who had been admitted with chest pain, and she didn't have time to check in with her friend. Susan had the day off, and it was only at the end of the shift that she managed to catch up with Gail.

"How was today?" she asked.

"I looked after that old lady again. She sure is demanding. Thank goodness her daughter is with her most of the time."

"Yes, it must be a real challenge to deal with someone like that all the time. Has she settled down yet?"

"Yes, she actually slept most of the afternoon, which is kind of nice. I gave her some medication after lunch, and it seemed to knock her right out. Her daughter managed to nap in the chair, too."

And then they reached their cars and they waved good-bye to each other. They both had one more shift, and then they had a couple of days off. Julie thought about her friend and the way she was dealing with everything. Gail was a strong woman, and she admired her a lot. I wonder how I would be if I had cancer, thought Julie, and then she shook her head as if to banish the thought. There but for the grace of God, she said silently to herself.

The next morning when they came on shift, the nursing manager was already on the unit. Rosemary was in her early thirties, a smart young woman who had risen in the corporate ranks quite quickly after joining the hospital. She could be a bit abrasive, and most of the nurses kept their distance from her. She was not one of them, and despite her relative youth, most of them were wary of her. She hardly ever came to the units, so her presence there, especially that early in the morning, meant that something bad had probably happened.

"Gail, can I see you for a moment?"

Gail had not even put her bag away in her locker. "Can I just put this away?" she replied.

"Why don't you bring it with you? We'll go to my office to talk."

The other nurses all looked at each other, their eyes wide with curiosity. It was not a good sign when the manager wanted to talk in her office. And why hadn't she allowed Gail to lock her bag away? Gail followed the manager down the hallway and toward the elevators. The contrast between the two of them was striking. The manager walked as if she were carrying a book on her head, and her heels made a clicking sound on the linoleum floor. Gail walked behind her, her shoulders slumped and the bottom of her scrub pants sweeping the floor. To the nurses on the unit, it was not a happy sight.

When they got to her office, the manager got right down to business. "Gail, it has come to my attention that you made an error when administering medication to a patient yesterday."

"What? When? Who?" Gail's words were jumbled together. She tried to remember how she could have made an error, but nothing came to mind.

"The patient is an elderly woman you admitted to the unit. It appears that you made a mistake in the dose of antipsychotic medication you gave her yesterday. The dose you gave her after lunch seems to be where the error was made. Do you recall how much was ordered for her and how much you gave?"

Gail stared at the woman across the desk. Her mind was blank, like a newly cleaned chalkboard. For the moment she could not remember anything about the elderly woman or about the medication she had given anyone.

"I'm not sure. I mean, I can't remember. I've never made a medication error before. Are you sure?"

"The patient's daughter complained to the night staff that her mother hadn't woken all afternoon. The medication orders were checked, and it appears that you gave her triple the dose. This is a very serious error. Fortunately the patient does not seem to have any lasting ill effects from the overdose, but the family is considering taking legal action. Can you explain how this might have happened?"

Tears flooded Gail's eyes, and she sat there, her shoulders slumped in defeat. She could barely look up and instead stared at her hands in her lap. How could this have happened? She was a good nurse, a careful nurse, and she had never made a mistake before. She didn't say anything. The two of them sat in uncomfortable silence for a few minutes. Then the manager started talking again.

"I have had reports from some of your colleagues that you are not quite yourself, Gail. They've noticed things and are worried about you."

———

Although there could be another reason for making an error when giving a patient medication, this may be another sign of cancer-related cognitive problems. Following written orders for giving medication requires organizational skills and executive functioning. Both of these can be affected by cognitive changes. Any alteration in one's ability to function normally can be both frustrating and frightening, but when it involves work-related issues, it can be very serious indeed.

Cognitive functioning may also be affected by cancer and its treatment in other ways: verbal memory (remembering words or things that have been read), motor functioning (using your hands to complete a task or misjudging the edge of a coffee table and dropping a cup), information processing (getting confused about what is being said to you), and language ability (having difficulty finding the right words).

———

Gail looked up at the manager, her face slack in disbelief. Tears had started to gather in her eyes, and as she sat there they ran down her face. She didn't have the energy to wipe them away, so she just let them run down either side of her nose and then off her chin.

"This is an awful situation, Gail. None of this is your fault, but I have a responsibility to our patients and to the rest of the staff. Until this is sorted out, you can't be at work."

Gail's face went white, and she felt dizzy. Not be at work! She wasn't sure she had heard properly. She had to be at work! She was a nurse, and she couldn't let her colleagues down. And then there was the issue of money. She had to work after all the time she had been off sick. She opened her mouth to speak, but no words came out. To her embarrassment, she felt a giant hiccup start in her throat, and she made a strangled noise as she tried to squash it.

The manager jumped in. "Gail, please listen to me. This is a safety issue, and as an organization we have to ensure that everyone is safe. We can't leave ourselves open to legal actions, and we can't allow that to happen to you, either. I have to make some arrangements this morning, but we want you to have some tests so that we can find out exactly what is going on and what can be done about it."

Rosemary continued to speak, but Gail didn't hear a word. She was staring at the young woman's face. She watched as her mouth opened and closed, opened and closed, her shiny lipstick catching the light from the fluorescent light fixture on the ceiling. The only way that Gail knew she was done talking was when she got up and put out her hand to touch Gail on the shoulder.

"What am I supposed to do now?" Gail asked quietly. She knew she had to say something, anything, to pretend that she had been listening.

"I think it's best if you went home right now. As soon as I have some information for you, I'll give you a call. Did you come by car this morning?"

Gail nodded.

"Well, then, I'll see if one of the secretaries can drive you home. You shouldn't be driving in this state."

"I'm fine. I don't want anyone to drive me home. I just need to be alone right now. I'm fine."

Gail pushed past the manager and ran down the hallway. She didn't care what she looked like or who could see her desperate flight down the hallway. She felt like such a failure! How could this have happened to her? She ran out of the hospital building and across the street to her car in the parking lot. She barely noticed the traffic, but she did hear the honking of horns as she ran across the road. When she got to the parking lot, she was momentarily confused. Where had she parked her car? Panic rose in her throat as she scanned the roofs of the hundreds of cars in their neat rows. For a moment she couldn't remember whose car she had driven to work, hers or Jim's. And where were her car keys? She patted the pockets of her uniform: nothing there! Then she realized that she still had her purse with her, and her keys were where she usually put them, in the outside pocket. Finding her keys calmed her a bit, and she saw her car under the big light stand in the spot where she always parked. She got in the car and sat for a few moments, her heart pounding. What was she going to do? How was she going to tell Jim? What were the other nurses going to think about her?

She drove home carefully, although when she pulled into the driveway she couldn't remember how she got there. The house was quiet when she turned the key in the lock, and she dropped her purse on the floor in the entrance hall. She just needed to think, so she went into the den and sat in her favorite chair. The next thing she knew, Jim was opening the door. Where had the time gone? He usually got home before her, and she could hear him calling her name as he put down his briefcase.

"Gail? Honey? You home? Is everything okay?"

She didn't answer. She just wanted to be able to keep what had happened away from him for a little bit longer. But he came into the den and saw her sitting in the chair.

"What happened? Why are you home already? Are you sick?" His voice was breathless with worry.

She opened her mouth to speak, and a loud sob broke out of her lungs. He immediately put his arms around her and let her cry, waiting patiently as he always did for her to stop and start talking. She told him what had happened in broken sentences, stopping frequently to draw in breath between her sobs. She told him about how difficult it was for her to concentrate and how she had made a medication error and how she had been told to go home. That was the worst of it for her. She had been sent home like a little child, and she didn't know how she was going to bear the shame.

Jim listened to all of this, his blue eyes never leaving her face. Every now and then he reached up with his hand and gently wiped the tears from her face. He didn't interrupt; he just kept his arms around her as she talked. She could sense that he was thinking about what she was telling him, and she so wanted him to tell her that everything was going to be okay. But he didn't say a word. When she finally stopped talking and crying, he hugged her against his chest.

"Honey, this may have been a blessing in disguise. Just hear me out now. You've been through a lot, but maybe you did go back to work before you should have. You put a lot of pressure on yourself, and I know you were worried about money. But here is an opportunity for you to make sure that you get well. This is not the end of the world."

Gail stiffened in his arms and pulled away from him. "How can you say that? This is my job you're talking about! They said I was not capable of doing my job!"

"It sounds like what they said is that you made an error and they want to cover their butts. You can surely understand why they have to do that. They have to make sure that you are okay to work. Did they tell you anything else?"

Gail suddenly remembered that Rosemary, the manager, had said something about having some tests. When she told Jim, his face changed. Had he noticed something?

"Honey, now, I want you to take this in the right way. You have been pretty forgetful in the last little while. I thought it would pass. I know how important your job is to you. And I also know that the last thing you would want is to put your patients in any kind of harm. So maybe these tests will be a good thing. Maybe they will show what you need to do to get better, to get over this finally."

He was right. She knew that. But it was still difficult to come to terms with. They were interrupted by the sound of the telephone. Jim went to answer and came back to the den with the phone in his hand.

"It's your manager. You have to talk to her."

He knew her so well. Rosemary was the last person she wanted to talk to at that moment. But Rosemary was calling to tell her that she needed to see her oncologist as soon as possible to discuss the possibility of a referral to a neurologist. Gail really liked her oncologist, a woman about her own age who worked at the cancer center affiliated with the hospital where she worked. Even though it was almost 4:00 p.m., Jim encouraged her to call to make an appointment. To her surprise, the nurse who worked with Dr. Lacey answered the phone. She didn't even ask why Gail wanted an appointment. She just told her to come in at the end of the day the following Monday.

"I'll come with you if you like." Jim's voice calmed her instantly.

Accepting this kind of bad news can be very challenging. We often have little insight into our own functioning, or we may be actively in denial about what is really going on. And often family members are reluctant to bring up problems for fear of upsetting someone they love. It is also often difficult to accept that things are not as they used to be or should be. People often find ways to compensate for forgetfulness, or the signs are so subtle that everyone around you makes allowances.

The next Monday, Gail and Jim went to see her oncologist. It had been five days since she was sent home from work, and the time had gone very slowly for her. She wasn't sure what to do with herself, and she wasted many hours just sitting in her chair and thinking. She was not sure what she had been thinking about, but she didn't have anything else to do and she couldn't remember what else she might have done.

Even though it was usually very busy in the cancer clinic, that day it was strangely quiet. And then Gail remembered that Dr. Lacey didn't usually have a Wednesday clinic. Perhaps she was being seen at a special time. That didn't make her feel any better, but she hardly had to wait at all. Almost as soon as they sat down, Gail heard her name called. They were ushered into one of the small family meeting rooms, a special room set aside for family conferences where people are usually told bad news. Gail felt her palms getting clammy, and she had to remind herself to breathe slowly. Jim just held her hand. The warmth from his palm helped her to remain focused.

Dr. Lacey entered the room after just a few minutes. She had Gail's chart in her hand, and she looked serious. "Hello, Gail. Hello, Jim. So, let's get started here. I received a call from your manager over at the hospital. She told me that you were having some difficulties. Can you tell me what has been going on?"

Gail felt her face go red. How dare Rosemary contact her oncologist and talk about her? She felt Jim's hand tighten over hers, and she pushed down her anger. She took a moment before she answered.

"Well, I made a mistake with a patient's medication. I've never made a mistake before! And I guess I have a hard time concentrating, especially in meetings. And I'm really tired. I don't sleep well, and that's probably why."

"Jim, have you noticed anything about Gail's overall functioning?"

Jim hesitated for a moment. He didn't want Gail to get upset, but this was an opportunity for her. So he took a deep breath and described what things had been like over the past few months. He talked about Gail being forgetful and how she sometimes just zoned out, often for long periods of time. He described her being at a loss for words quite often. Gail sat there, a ball of something rising in her throat. Why had Jim not said anything? How could he have kept all these things from her? Her thoughts came to an abrupt stop when she heard Dr. Lacey say her name loudly.

"Gail? What do you think?"

"Um, I don't know. I'm just so tired all the time. I guess I have been a bit forgetful, too. I don't know. I just don't know what to do or think or feel!"

"This sounds like it may be related to your treatment. You have a few options that I am going to tell you about, so I need you to concentrate. Can you stick with me for a few minutes?"

Gail nodded, and Jim pulled a small notebook out of his pocket. He sat with a pen in his hand, and Gail felt so grateful for this sensible husband of hers who was always prepared.

"We now know that some patients get something that we used to call chemo-brain. But it's not just from chemotherapy. These brain changes can be due to all sorts of things. We can try you on a medication that seems to help with memory and concentration. Or we can see if it is your antiestrogen medication that is causing the problems."

Gail was stunned. Why had no one told her about this? In all the time she had been a patient, no one had even mentioned that any of her treatments could cause changes in her brain. Her mind was whirling with questions, but before she could say anything, Jim stepped in.

"Shouldn't she have some sort of testing to see what's happening, Dr. Lacey? It seems strange to offer treatment without knowing what the cause is."

"Well, the fact of the matter is that we don't really have any definitive test for this. So we mostly try to deal with it by giving medication or perhaps by taking away the antiestrogen medication."

There are a number of tests available to identify specific areas where cognition is altered. But the tests are not very accurate, and the results can be difficult to interpret. Knowing the area affected unfortunately does not provide clear interventions for treatment, either. It is suggested that listening to the patient's reported symptoms rather than relying on tests is the best way to go with the present level of knowledge in this area.

There is also little evidence about the role of antiestrogens in this phenomenon. However, women on this medication often report changes in mood, their ability to concentrate, and memory, so stopping the medication may be a good first step. If cognitive functioning improves, then a cause may have been found. Of course, a challenge of this approach is that the woman then needs to go on another drug (such as an aromatase inhibitor) to reduce the risk of recurrence of breast cancer.

There is some evidence that a psychostimulant called methylphenidate is useful in the treatment of cancer-related cognitive changes. This medication is commonly used to treat attention-deficit hyperactivity disorder. Like any other medication, it can have significant side effects, but studies in women with cancer have shown benefits.

It has also been suggested that because cognitive changes are so common after treatment for cancer, the risk for this should be part of the consent process before someone starts treatment. This approach has not gained significant support, so patients are often not warned that cognitive changes may occur.

"That's a lot to take in, Dr. Lacey." Jim's careful words helped Gail feel calm, when what she really wanted to do was bolt out of the room.

"I know. I want Gail to have some time to think about this. There are also some other things she can do. There are all sorts of ways that she can help herself—making lists, setting reminders. One or two of my patients have consulted with an occupational therapist, and this has been helpful to them."

There has been a lot of research on helping the elderly with cognitive decline, and many of these strategies can be helpful for the person with cancer-related cognitive changes. Merely knowing that the changes are due to the cancer or its treatment can be reassuring. People often think they are going crazy, and reassurance can help them start adapting to the changes.

These changes are not related to other neurological conditions that are progressive (such as Alzheimer's disease) and do not indicate any change in the recovery from cancer. They are also not related to the recurrence of cancer.

Strategies for coping with these challenges include using written reminders of tasks to be accomplished, using an electronic device such as a digital diary to send audible alerts when tasks have to be performed, and keeping a detailed calendar of events with sticky notes that can be removed and carried to act as reminders.

Exercise has been shown to help as well. It improves strength and stamina and promotes oxygenation of the brain. Reducing or eliminating background noise and limiting concurrent multiple tasks can also help concentration. Doing intellectually stimulating activities such as crossword puzzles and sudoku can help exercise the brain and has been shown to maintain brain activity in the elderly.

"What would happen to me if I stopped the antiestrogen? I thought you said it would cut my risk of recurrence, so what would happen if I stopped it?" Gail seemed to have found her voice.

"Well, we would put you on another medication to lower your risk of recurrence. You would normally go on that medication after five years of antiestrogens, so we are just getting you a head start on that. You may find that if you stop the antiestrogen, your hot flashes will stop and your sleep may get better."

"Then that's what I want to do. How soon would I see results?"

"You may notice some changes quite quickly. I would still encourage you to see the occupational therapist, but . . ."

"I'll think about that. But I need to get better quickly so that I can get back to work. Jim, don't say a word!"

Jim had opened his mouth to suggest that she take some time to think about it. But she seemed so decisive that he shut it again. It really was her decision to make, and in a way he was happy to see her take charge of something.

"Okay. So I'll just get you a prescription for the aromatase inhibitor. I'd like to see you again in about a month to see how you're doing."

"Can I go back to work now?"

Dr. Lacey hesitated. "It's not for me to say when you should go back to work. You need to talk to your manager about that. But I will tell her that we have changed your medication, and that might help."

Gail was impatient as she waited for Dr. Lacey to come back into the room with her prescription. Jim decided to just wait it out. She would talk when she was ready. Something had changed in his wife. He could tell by the way she held her shoulders. She was mad, and that seemed to push aside the despondency he had seen in her since she was sent home from work. He privately thought that seeing the occupational therapist was a great idea, but he knew better than to contradict his wife when she was mad. It took Dr. Lacey just a few minutes to write the prescription, and she handed it over along with a business card for the occupational therapist. Gail glanced at the card briefly and then put it in her pants pocket. She quickly read over the prescription, thanked the oncologist, and motioned with her head to Jim that it was time to leave. On the way home, they stopped at the drug store, and Gail went in with the prescription clutched tightly in her hand.

When they got home, Jim watched as Gail went into the bathroom and closed the door. He heard a loud noise as something landed in the garbage can. She must have thrown away the bottle of antiestrogen medication. Jim smiled. That was so like the old Gail who used to be decisive and focused. Perhaps it really would help, and as he thought about it, he decided that he was going to will it to happen. He was also going to help her in any way he could. If that meant he had to call her to remind her of what she had to do on the way home, then he would do that. And if he had to take on extra responsibilities at home, then he would do that, too.

Her mood seemed brighter at dinner that night. He didn't feel like warming up soup, their usual dinner, and he wanted to mark the occasion in some way. So he ordered in some pizza and a salad and set the table with the good silverware and linen napkins. Gail smiled when she saw how much trouble he'd gone to, and even though she was still worried about their finances, she didn't say anything about the expense. They ate in comfortable silence, each deep in thought about the events of the day and what might happen in the future.

The next morning, Gail called Rosemary, the manager of the unit at the hospital. Even though she thought she had planned what she was going to say, as she listened to the sound of the phone ringing in her ear, she almost panicked. She had written down her main points, and she wanted to be sure she stuck to them and didn't get sidetracked.

"Rosemary Voight." The manager's greeting was crisp when she eventually answered the phone.

"Hello. This is Gail, Gail Summers. You know, the nurse from 5A." Gail felt herself losing momentum even with her greeting.

"Yes, hello, Gail. How are you?"

"Well, better I think. Um, I wanted to talk to you about . . ."

She quickly checked her notes, where she had written in large uppercase letters the words "arrange a meeting."

"I would like to come in and talk to you about my return to work." That was better. Even to her own ears she sounded confident and assured.

"Isn't this a bit early?" Rosemary sounded like she wanted to take control of the phone call.

"Well, it may seem early to you, but it has been six days since you sent me home. I've seen my oncologist, and I want to talk to you about returning to work."

There! She'd said it. She felt proud of herself for that. She'd managed to get the words out, and she hadn't been intimidated. Well, just a little bit.

"Okay, then. I'm going to have to get someone from human resources to be at the meeting, so I have to contact them first. But I do have some time on Thursday morning, around ten o'clock. I'll ask someone from HR to be here for that. I'll call to reschedule if that's not possible. Good-bye, Gail."

It was only Tuesday, so she had forty-eight hours to wait before the meeting. She decided she would make a list of all the things she did during a shift to see if she could identify areas where she might need help. The list was long: helping patients to bathe, taking vital signs, giving out medication, talking to the physicians, checking on the orders they wrote, talking to the patients' families, preparing the patients for tests and procedures, and explaining those tests and procedures to the patients and their families. She wasn't sure she had covered everything, but it was a start. She rewrote the list, this time making sure that her handwriting was neat. She left space on the right-hand side of the page where she could make notes. She ticked the tasks that she thought she could do without much help. The list helped her to feel more in control, and she put it carefully in the side pocket of her purse where she would be sure to have it with her for the meeting with Rosemary.

———

Making lists is a useful way of identifying what needs to be done. It also helps to break down what may seem to be a complex set of actions into smaller, more manageable steps. Many people use lists for all sorts of things: to be reminded of what they have to do, to weigh the pros and cons of a certain action, and to help them focus on details. For Gail, making a list of her tasks during a typical shift may help her to persuade her manager of what she can do as opposed to what she can't.

———

When she woke up on Thursday morning, Gail realized that she had slept through the whole night without any disruptions. As she thought about it, she realized that she had not had a hot flash since she stopped the medication. She sat on the edge of the bed, feeling really rested and refreshed after a night's sleep for the first time in ages. Maybe going off the antiestrogen medication was helping! She entered the bathroom where Jim was shaving with a spring in her step.

"Do you notice anything different about me?"

Jim hesitated, his razor in his hand and half of his face covered in white cream. "You look as lovely as you usually do first thing in the morning!" was his response.

Gail laughed. "Flattery will get you bonus points, but I'm serious. Can you notice anything different?"

Jim looked at his wife's reflection in the mirror. There was something about her this morning, but he was not sure what it was. She hadn't showered yet, and her hair was flat on one side and matted on the other.

"I slept through the whole night! I didn't wake up once! No hot flashes. Not even one!" Her voice was triumphant.

"That's great, honey. You must feel so . . ." He was not sure what to say after that.

"I feel rested, Jim, really rested. It's like I had the best night's sleep of my whole life. It's kind of like what happened when the kids started sleeping through the night when they were babies. I feel alive! Like I can do anything!"

Jim decided not to say anything that would ruin the moment for her. He was not sure what was happening, but if one night of good sleep made this kind of difference, he was really happy. Gail quickly got into the shower, and the small bathroom filled with the sound of her humming as the water flowed over her. She had not sung in the shower for a very long time. In fact, he was not sure that she even showered every day anymore. The sound of her humming over the sound of the water felt normal, blissfully normal to him, and he resumed his shave with a smile on his face.

They ate breakfast together, not talking much as Jim looked over the newspaper and Gail emptied the dishwasher in between bites of her toast. She lifted her head so that he could kiss her cheek, and then he was gone and she was left alone with her thoughts about her meeting with Rosemary and the person from HR later that morning. She shook her head and reminded herself that she was feeling good that day, and she was not going to let her fears take away that feeling. She left early for the meeting, concerned about finding a parking spot in the lot. She considered stopping by the unit to say hello to the other nurses but thought better of it. She wanted to get this meeting with Rosemary over and done with. Perhaps she would go by the unit after the meeting. She was twenty minutes early, and she was worried that if she sat waiting for Rosemary, she would get all nervous. So she sat in her car, reading over the list she had made describing what she did during her shift.

She managed to stay in her car for only ten more minutes and then walked slowly from the parking lot to the hospital. It felt strange to be walking through the doors and not to be going on shift. Even her street clothes felt odd. She always wore scrubs to work, and she missed their familiar softness and comfort. When she got to Rosemary's office, she found that the person from HR was already waiting. They smiled at each other, and Gail immediately felt at ease. The woman introduced herself as Bonnie Bartlett, and Gail remembered that she had attended a session this woman had done on investing for retirement. She had used a lot of humor in that presentation and had put the audience at ease. Maybe this would not be that bad!

At exactly ten o'clock, Rosemary opened the door of her office. She seemed surprised that the two of them were outside waiting. She ushered them into her office, and as she started speaking, Bonnie interrupted her.

"Rosemary, if you don't mind, I would like to start this meeting by telling Gail that we are here to support her and not to punish her. Employees are often really anxious about these kinds of meetings, and I want Gail to know that we are here to help her come back to work as safely and quickly as possible. Like all our employees, Gail is a valuable asset, and we would hate for her to think that she is not important to the organization. Now please go ahead and say what you wanted to say."

There was an awkward silence as Rosemary searched for something to say. Gail felt her shoulders relax, and she jumped in. "Thank you, Bonnie. That means a lot to me. I love my work and have always tried to be the best nurse I could be. I went to see my oncologist on Monday, and we came up with a plan to change my medication. I know it's early, but I can already feel the difference. When can I come back?"

———※———

Gail may be overly optimistic about her improvement off the medication. Real change may take a month or more. But just getting some decent sleep can make a world of difference. The supportive comments of the HR person have put her at ease, and being able to think and talk without pressure and fear can really help a person feel confident and think clearly.

———※———

Rosemary seemed to be quite taken aback by how the meeting was going. She sat in her chair, blinking her eyes as if trying to regain control. "I thought that perhaps we could talk about what Gail would need to do before she could come back."

"How about we rephrase that?" Bonnie's voice was soft and slow, but her meaning was clear. This was going to be a positive and supportive meeting despite the tactic that Rosemary seemed to want to take. "How can we make this an easy transition for Gail? What can we do to help her?"

"I made a list of all the things I would do in an average shift, and I marked the ones where I think I would be just fine. I know there are other areas where I need some help, mostly getting organized and remembering stuff, and I would be happy to have any help with that. I'm finding that making lists helps, as long as I can remember where I put the lists."

Bonnie's laughter filled the office. "We have a lot in common, Gail! I'm always losing my shopping lists! This looks like a good start, and I'm glad that you've been so proactive. Now Rosemary, what do you think?"

Rosemary looked like she had a lot of thoughts in her head, but she gave in gracefully. She reached over and took Gail's list and started reading.

"I think we can work with this. How about you come back, starting on Monday, and we'll buddy you with someone? That way there'll be someone to help you with meds and teaching, someone to check in with if you're not sure. And maybe for the first couple of weeks we can have you on a reduced work week, maybe half time until you are sure you can manage. Does that sound okay?"

It sounded more than okay to Gail. It sounded like the warmest "welcome home" she had ever heard. She felt the knots in her neck and shoulders give way to a warm feeling, and she smiled with her mouth and her eyes and her heart. She was coming home.

Part III

SURVIVING AND THRIVING: THE NEW NORMAL

• 11 •

A Blueprint for Health

$\mathscr{A}$fter reading the stories of the nine cancer survivors in part II, what are the most important take-home messages for living well in the new normal? From a review of the literature and from working with many cancer survivors, there are nine fundamental issues facing cancer survivors. This chapter highlights the most important aspects of thriving during the many years of survivorship.

1. FEAR OF RECURRENCE

Many cancer survivors will tell you that life is never the same after diagnosis and treatment. What was once normal and could be taken for granted is just not there anymore. Cancer changes everything, and life is now experienced as a new normal. Something else that is very common is the fear of the cancer coming back. This fear of recurrence may never leave the survivor. It may become easier to manage, and the survivor may have hours or days or weeks when they don't think about the cancer. But any change in how they feel physically (a new cough, a sudden pain) brings one thought to the forefront: is the cancer back?

Some cancer survivors experience intrusive thoughts. These are thoughts, usually of a painful or frightening nature, that pop into your head. They seem to occur quite randomly, with no specific prompt. They can cause physical symptoms such as faster heartbeat and rapid breathing; they can even cause a panic attack.

One of the characteristics of intrusive thoughts and feelings is that they are not realistic or logical. They tend to spiral out of control until they lead you to a situation of pure panic. It is quite common that these fears center on coping with everyday activities and responsibilities. For women, these thoughts often involve how they would have to rely on other people to take care of their family and home responsibilities if the cancer came back.

So, what can you do to help control your thoughts? Keeping a diary and refocusing your thoughts are two strategies that may be helpful for people who find that they are having anxiety-provoking thoughts and feelings. It requires commitment and attention and may not be right for everyone. When keeping a diary, you should note the stressful event (such as having to go to the cancer center for follow-up care), and then you should note what it was about the event that made it stressful or anxiety provoking; what your physical and emotional reactions were to the event (for example, your heart beating faster); how intense these reactions were; how you handled the event; and what you would do differently the next time.

Connected with this is the strategy of refocusing your thoughts. For example, if you have to go to the cancer center for follow-up care, on the way there you might start thinking about the bad news you may hear at your appointment. Your thoughts may turn to what would happen if the cancer is back. So your initial thought, "They are going to tell me that the cancer is back," is replaced with a refocused thought, "I am just going for my regular follow-up appointment. I have not experienced any symptoms that suggest the cancer is back." When you first start doing this, it may feel forced. But the more often you do it, the easier and more natural it will feel. The intent is not to make you happy all the time, but rather to help you avoid negative thinking and instead think more positively and realistically.

So, what else can be done to control these irrational fears? Being part of a support group that focuses on problem solving or stress reduction may help. Such groups are more effective in reducing anxiety and depression and in improving quality of life than support groups with little focus.

Support groups can be a good source of both information and support. There are different kinds of support groups, and it may take a while to find one that best meets your needs. Some support groups are disease specific (for example, a support group for women with breast cancer). Some are age specific. Some support groups encourage partners and family members to attend, while others are only for patients and survivors. There is usually a facilitator for the support group, and this person may be a professional, such as a social worker, or a layperson, such as another cancer survivor.

It is important to judge whether what is discussed at the support group meetings is valuable to you. Some support groups are focused on sharing information and have a guest speaker at each meeting. Other support groups are less focused, and those attending are free to talk about whatever they want. Sometimes these sorts of support groups turn into a gripe session about things that are not very constructive. It is also important to keep in mind that the experiences of other survivors in a group may not necessarily translate to your experience. If you find that attending a support group makes you more worried or depressed, then perhaps you need to find another support group or to stop attending one entirely.

It can be very difficult to admit that you need help coping after cancer treatment. It is especially difficult to do when you are months or even years after treatment and you assume that you should be feeling like your old self. Many survivors believe they have to think and act and feel a certain way and not complain. They may even be given the message that they should just be happy to have survived when others have not.

Finding and accepting help is a big hurdle to overcome. Many people resist seeking help because they think it means they are weak. We live in a society where there is a push-pull between the expectation of being so self-sufficient that you never ask for help and the helplessness of some people who seem unable to figure things out for themselves and constantly seek support and even medication.

Something else that can help is to find ways to consciously relax and prevent the physical sensations of fear and anxiety. Progressive muscle relaxation is a simple technique to learn and can help reduce stress and anxiety. Detailed instructions are provided in chapter 12. Deep breathing can also help with these relaxation exercises, or it can be done by itself. It may sound silly to have to learn how to breathe, but most of us don't do it properly. So a few minutes of instruction can start a lifetime of better breathing!

Mindfulness-based stress reduction is a form of meditation and yoga that has been shown to significantly improve mood and quality of life. The focus of mindfulness meditation is on being present in the moment without getting distracted by memories of the past or anticipation about the future. The intention is not to bring about relaxation, but relaxation often does occur as a side effect of the meditation. There are four kinds of mindfulness practice: awareness of sensation, sitting meditation, body scan, and mindful movement. A full description is presented in chapter 12.

It is important to remember that no technique or intervention will help immediately. These things take time and patience and commitment. But they do not involve taking pills or experiencing side effects, and they may be a good place to start on your own. It's a matter of finding something that you can do regularly and to which you are willing to commit.

2. DEPRESSION

The end of treatment is a milestone for most people with cancer. The weeks and months of going to the hospital or cancer center are over, and many patients think they should celebrate this in some way. But often there is little to celebrate. At the end of treatment, most people are at their weakest physically and often emotionally, too. This is a time when the side effects of treatment are often at their worst. It is not uncommon for the person with cancer to experience depression when treatment ends.

Probably the most notable difference for patients is that they don't have to go for treatment anymore, and this leaves a lot of empty hours in the days and weeks ahead. As much as treatment can be difficult, there is also comfort in knowing that you are being well cared for. Seeing the nurses and physicians regularly makes many people feel safe. They know that they are being monitored and that the nurses and physicians will take care of any problems that occur. Many patients become very attached to their health care providers, and the end of treatment feels almost like a breakup of a relationship. Being at home alone after the intense period of treatment may feel lonely and strange, and most people are not prepared for this.

Part of the transition out of active treatment means letting go of the relationships that were formed as part of the treatment, and this can be very challenging for some patients. There is even a term for this: *deprofessionalizing*, which means reducing the amount of care-seeking behavior. But for most patients it can feel like loss or abandonment.

There are some classic signs of depression: feelings of sadness, lack of pleasure in life (anhedonia), hopelessness and helplessness, low self-esteem and low self-worth, feelings of guilt, and suicidal thoughts. Another important sign of depression is difficulty sleeping. These are not unusual in the cancer survivor, and some studies estimate that up to 25 percent of people with cancer experience depression. Age, gender, type and stage of cancer, and the presence of social support all affect how often depression occurs, and depression can be experienced anywhere in the cancer journey, from diagnosis to the end of life. It is not unusual for depression to occur after treatment is over. Given what we know about all the attention and busyness involved in the fight for survival during cancer treatment, it is easy to see how people can get depressed when the treatment is over.

The role of the cancer patient is quite clearly defined: you have to fight the cancer with all your energy, and you give yourself over to being taken care of by efficient and caring health care providers. Then you get through with the treatment, and then . . . well, then what? People around you may assume that after active treatment is over, you go right back to being the person you were before. But how can you be the same as you were before? You may assume that you have to get back to the old you, and you may have an unrealistic timetable for doing that.

We know that depression can profoundly affect quality of life for the cancer survivor. And it can also increase the risk of relapse after treatment. Some studies suggest that depression can even affect survival. These are serious consequences, so depression should be identified early and treated. Some cancer care providers routinely ask patients and survivors if they are feeling depressed or are showing other signs of distress (depression is a sign of emotional distress). They may use screening tools (a brief questionnaire, for example) at every visit or ask the person if he or she is feeling sad or is not sleeping well. Others don't ask about this and may even assume that depression is a normal part of the cancer experience.

It is not easy to admit that you are depressed. Sometimes it's even harder to admit it to someone you love. A big part of depression may be your inability to get motivated enough to ask for help or to describe how you are feeling. People cope in different ways, and how you cope in general may predict your likelihood of becoming depressed. For example, if you tend to be less optimistic in your overall outlook, you may be more likely to become depressed after cancer treatment is over. If you use denial as a coping mechanism, you are also more likely to become depressed after treatment. People who have any kind of difficulty with everyday activities are also more likely to be depressed after treatment. And if you have problems with depression before cancer treatment, you are even more likely to be depressed afterward. It can be very difficult to ask for help or even to accept help when it is offered.

Some cancer survivors have the typical signs of posttraumatic stress disorder, like those seen in people who have experienced some kind of traumatic event. The symptoms of this for people with cancer include reliving certain treatments, experiencing difficulties getting to sleep and staying asleep, nightmares, and difficulties resuming normal relationships. This can be treated with counseling and also with antidepressant medication. If it is not treated, the person may experience significant challenges in making the transition from cancer patient to cancer survivor.

Cognitive behavioral therapy (a kind of talk therapy) has been shown to be effective in treating depression, and many psychiatrists offer a combination of medication and counseling. Some people find support groups helpful. There is increasing evidence that exercise can have a beneficial effect on mood, but this has not been tested extensively in people with cancer.

Many people are a little afraid of counseling. They assume that they are going to have to tell all their deep, dark secrets. But often counseling shows us how our thoughts and feelings interact with our behavior. It can be very useful in changing how we think about events and for finding a more positive outlook on life or dealing with difficult situations. It has been shown to be very effective in treating depression, insomnia, and different kinds of anxiety disorders.

3. GOING BACK TO WORK

There are over ten million cancer survivors in the United States today. An estimated 3.8 million of them are adults who were employed at the time of their diagnosis and return to work after treatment, and some may even have worked throughout their treatment. Continuing to work is important for financial reasons, but also for self-esteem and social support. Returning to work is symbolic of having gotten through treatment and of a return to normality and stability. Many cancer survivors have to work to retain health insurance coverage, although their diagnosis may cause problems in that regard. On the other hand, a life-altering diagnosis can also prompt a reevaluation of priorities. Some people may choose to leave a job they do not enjoy to seek more satisfying employment, or they may take early retirement and focus on family and leisure activities instead of work.

It may not be smooth sailing, however. Employers may assume that someone with cancer is no longer capable of carrying out their work as well as they did before. This may lead to discrimination, both subtle and overt, and cancer survivors have reported being dismissed, passed over for promotion, and denied benefits, as well as having experienced hostility in the workplace. All of these contravene the Americans with Disabilities Act (ADA), which was passed in 1990. People with cancer are included under this protection because cancer is regarded as a disease that impairs or limits a major life activity. The law, however, does not provide blanket coverage, and whether an employee is covered is decided on a case-by-case basis. Some courts have identified a weakness in the law: if a person with cancer is well enough to want to work, then they are not considered disabled.

Under the Americans with Disabilities Act, an employer with more than fifteen employees must make reasonable accommodation for workers with a disability, as long as this does not impose an "undue hardship" on the company's business. Undue hardship is defined as anything that requires significant difficulty or expense in light of the company's size or resources. The employer is also not required to lower quality or production standards in making the accommodation or to provide personal-use items such as hearing aids for an employee.

The ADA prohibits discrimination in hiring or firing employees and in the provision of benefits. Reasonable accommodations that should be made for employees with cancer include changes in work hours or time off for medical appointments and side effects from treatment. Most accommodations for workers do not cost money, and if they do, the amount is usually very little, around $500.

The Family and Medical Leave Act (FMLA) applies to companies with over fifty employees. Under this act, the company must allow twelve weeks of unpaid leave for an employee during any twelve-month period, and it requires the company to continue to provide benefits, including health insurance, during the leave period. The employee must be allowed to return to the same or an equivalent position after the leave. FMLA also allows leave to care for a spouse, child, or parent with a serious health condition and for a reduced work schedule when medically necessary.

There are different ways of planning a return to work. The kind of work plays a role, as does how well the recovery from treatment is progressing. We know that people who do physical work, particularly if there is heavy lifting involved, often have a more difficult time returning to work.

It is important to start making plans *before* your sick leave is over. Although it is important to get the "all clear" from your treating physician, it is also important to consult someone who understands the issues related to the work you do. An occupational health specialist can be very helpful in this regard. Your company or insurance plan may have someone you can speak to before you go back to work. An occupational health specialist will usually assess your physical and emotional health and ask questions about the kind of work you do, the work environment, and other factors that may impact your return to work.

It is helpful to have a plan in writing that you draw up with your supervisor in consultation with the occupational health specialist. The plan needs to clearly describe how many hours you can work, the kind of work you will be doing, how your work hours will increase over time if you are on a graduated back-to-work program, and the proposed date when you will be back at work or working full time. This plan should be evaluated with your supervisor every two weeks and adjusted as needed. You may be able to speed up the plan, or you may have to alter it to allow more time on a reduced workload. If the plan is not working for you or your supervisor, you may have to draw up a revised work plan that is more realistic. It is also important to let your coworkers know that you are on a back-to-work plan so that they will understand that you are not slacking off but rather are working reduced hours for a certain period of time or have made adjustments to your role. Transparency can prevent a lot of problems.

Work is important to most of us, and returning to work is often seen as a marker of recovery and surviving the cancer. Trying to make this milestone easy and problem free is an important task for the cancer survivor.

4. FATIGUE

Fatigue is a common side effect of cancer treatment and one that often comes as a surprise when it persists after treatment is over. There is no timetable for recovery from the fatigue, and many people get very frustrated when the tiredness drags on for weeks and months. There has been a fair amount of study into managing cancer-related fatigue. Some interventions have been shown to work, while others have yet to prove their effectiveness. Exercise is the only intervention that has been shown in studies to help with cancer-related fatigue.

Sleep quality can affect energy levels during the day. Getting a good night's sleep can really help, but the converse is true, too. Poor sleep is a significant contributor to fatigue. Some strategies that have been shown to improve sleep are avoiding late-afternoon or long naps; limiting time in bed to actual sleeping instead of watching TV in bed before sleep; going to bed only when sleepy; setting a consistent time for going to sleep and waking up; avoiding caffeine, sodas, and other stimulants in the evening; and establishing a presleep routine that is practiced consistently.

Here are some interventions that may be helpful in the management of treatment-related fatigue: Screen for causes of the fatigue, and manage those as appropriate. Conserving energy and altering one's activities to manage fatigue may also be helpful. Balancing rest and activity can help, but the person may have to ask others to help with this, and not everyone has that kind of support or is willing to ask for it. Relaxation exercises, massage, and healing touch may also help, although there is less evidence that these are effective.

There have been some studies investigating the use of medication to treat cancer-related fatigue. The medications tested were mostly stimulants or antidepressants, and although they were helpful for some people, they also had significant side effects, and experts suggest that the risks may outweigh the benefits.

Exercise helps in many different ways to improve one's quality of life and level of functioning. It can help lower the risk of heart disease and osteoporosis, improve balance, lower the risk for depression and anxiety, help with weight control, improve sleep, and combat fatigue. It is important to do the kind of exercise that you enjoy and to customize it so that you can do it with comfort and without compromising your safety. Some people really like to go to the gym and work up a good sweat. This may not be possible soon after completing treatments that have left you weak with and perhaps some challenges keeping your balance. You may need the help of a specialist such as a physiotherapist or an exercise trainer to help you modify your exercise routine.

Getting started with an exercise plan is just the first step. It is much harder to keep at it, and there are three simple steps that will help you stick to your plan. The first is to set realistic goals. The second is to reward yourself when you are consistent in actually doing whatever exercise you have planned. And the third is to establish a support system that will validate what you are doing and support you in your plan. Slow and steady should be the mantra. No matter what exercise you do, you should be able to talk in full sentences without getting short of breath. If you cannot do that, your intensity is too high, and you need to slow down.

A realistic goal is important because you will only succeed if you can actually do what you have planned. Attempting to do too much will result in frustration and will use up energy instead of creating energy. Rewarding yourself is important too, because a reward provides motivation to continue and be persistent. A reward can be anything that feels like a treat: a nice bar of soap that you would not usually buy, a new best-seller, or a movie rental. Having a support system, a person or group of people who encourages you and helps you achieve your exercise goals, can go a long way toward ensuring that you keep up with your plans and goals. Someone who exercises with you can be really helpful, because on any day that you are thinking about not exercising, knowing that you are letting someone else down can be a powerful motivation to just do it!

5. SEXUALITY

Changes in sexuality and sexual functioning are a common but often neglected side effect of cancer and its treatment. It is typical for both men and women to lose interest in sex as part of the cancer experience. From diagnosis through treatment, sex may disappear altogether as the person faces multiple diagnostic tests and various treatments. However, some couples find that being sexual provides a welcome relief from stress, and they may actually be more sexual in the face of a life-threatening illness.

Many people do not feel any interest in sex while undergoing chemotherapy or radiation or after surgery. It is important to check with a health care provider if precautions need to be taken to prevent chemotherapy agents from affecting a partner if body fluids are exchanged. It is often necessary to use condoms to prevent the partner from coming in contact with semen or vaginal secretions that may contain by-products of the chemotherapy. For people who have depressed immune systems from chemotherapy, it may be best to avoid sexual contact altogether to reduce the risk of infection.

Chemotherapy often puts women into an early menopause, and some women never see the return of their normal menstrual cycle. The ovaries shut down and stop producing hormones, resulting in hot flashes and a dry and painful vagina. Estrogen is a female hormone that, among other things, keeps the tissues of the vagina moist and healthy. It is sometimes called the hormone of arousal because of its effects on vaginal lubrication. Many women find vaginal penetration painful after menopause, and it may be even more difficult for women who go into instant menopause from chemotherapy instead of the gradual decline in hormones experienced during natural menopause.

Radiation therapy can affect sexuality in different ways, too. The fatigue that is often a major side effect of this kind of treatment may push thoughts of sex right out of the mind of the person undergoing treatment. Depending on where the cancer is and where the beams of radiation are aimed, further side effects may make sexual touch or intercourse difficult. Women with breast cancer may experience skin irritation over the chest wall. Radiation to the pelvis may result in difficulties achieving and maintaining erections for men or vaginal dryness and shortening for women.

Surgery to remove the prostate, bladder, or rectum in men tends to have a profound effect on erections, as the nerves that cause erections may be damaged or destroyed. Surgery for bladder, gynecological, or colon cancer in women can also destroy nerves and cause changes in the structure and function of the pelvic anatomy, making sex painful or even impossible.

Cancer survivors report that this topic is often neglected during treatment and into the recovery stage. Some health care providers find this a difficult topic to talk about and so do not raise it with their patients. And if the health care provider doesn't talk about it, the patient often feels that it is not something that should be talked about. This is a great pity, as sexuality is an important part of quality of life, and many couples find that it is not easy to solve sexual problems on their own.

It can be surprisingly easy to slip into the habit of not talking and not touching one's spouse or partner. Although some couples are happy to live in a sexless relationship, lack of sex can lead to a lack of emotional closeness, as well as sexual frustration. It can be quite difficult to change this pattern, and as the days and weeks and months go by, the distance makes it even more difficult to start a conversation about what is happening to the relationship. Some couples find themselves arguing more, while others just drift further and further apart.

Sexual problems can be the spark for much bitterness because sex represents different things to different people. Either partner can see lack of sex as personal rejection, and this can hurt very deeply. It is also possible that one person may assume things that are not true. However, if they don't talk about it, these assumptions become an insurmountable barrier because the other person may not even know what the original assumptions were.

Marital therapy or couple's counseling can be an effective way to resolve differences and get the couple talking to one another in a meaningful way. The counselor or therapist can control the conversation and prompt positive ways of resolving conflict. But both partners have to engage in the process, and when one withholds or refuses to participate, it can be difficult. A skilled therapist or counselor can usually elicit a lot of information with carefully worded questions. Often the person has not thought about the problem from all angles, and this skillful questioning can provide the person with solutions that come from within.

Some people are not sure what a sex therapist actually does, and there are many misconceptions about sex therapy in general. A sex therapist is a highly educated professional who is usually certified, most often by the American Association of Sex Educators, Counselors and Therapists (www.AASECT .org). Sex therapists may specialize in one particular area (for example, working with couples who are dealing with chronic illness) or may see a wide range of couples and single people who are experiencing sexual difficulties. Sex therapy usually involves talking about the problem and figuring out what might help. It does *not* involve nudity or having sex in front of the counselor.

6. EXERCISE AND DIET

Many people with cancer attempt to make changes in their diet and amount of exercise. Not only is it challenging to make lifestyle changes, but it is even more difficult to sustain them in the long run. People need all the help and support they can get, and having a loving and involved family is a definite asset. Studies show that cancer survivors do make lifestyle changes. In one large study, almost 92 percent of survivors did not smoke, and almost half got regular exercise, but less than 20 percent ate the recommended five servings of fruit and vegetables a day. Only 5 percent of cancer survivors in this study met all three recommendations.

There is increasing evidence that obesity and cancer are linked, although the precise nature of the link is not clear. Obesity has been shown to adversely affect a cancer prognosis, so it is very important that anyone with a cancer diagnosis maintain a healthy weight for their height. In addition, obesity causes many other health problems such as diabetes and heart disease, and these remain significant threats to overall health and well-being outside of the risks of cancer. Other risks to health come from smoking, drinking alcohol, and a lack of physical activity. Although what you eat won't cure cancer, a good diet may help you stay healthy and can help you regain strength, fight infection, and feel better. It is important to eat a varied diet with a focus on plant-based foods. Colorful fruits and vegetables contain the most nutrients. Whole grains and legumes are good sources of complex carbohydrates and fiber. Consume less than one cup of lean protein and low-fat dairy products a day. Minimize your intake of fat, salt, sugar, alcohol, and smoked or pickled foods. Steam, boil, or poach your foods instead of frying or charbroiling. Making lifestyle changes such as improving diet and increasing exercise can make a significant difference in quality of life for cancer survivors, especially for those who are older or overweight.

Recommendations from the American Cancer Society, the Centers for Disease Control and Prevention, the American College of Sports Medicine, and the World Health Organization advise cancer survivors to participate in moderate exercise for thirty minutes or more at least five days a week. Survivors should get the approval of their oncologist before starting an exercise program, and if there is a risk that long-term effects of cancer treatment may affect the cardiovascular system, then assessment and screening should be done first to ensure that the survivor is healthy enough. Some larger cancer centers have rehabilitation programs where survivors can participate in exercise in a managed setting where their overall well-being can be monitored.

Although initiating lifestyle changes may not be easy, it is often more difficult to maintain the changes over the long term. As the novelty of the new behavior wears off, some may find that their commitment decreases, and they slip back into old habits. Family and friends can be great motivators and supporters. But it is a long process, one that you should follow for the rest of your life, and the temptation to stop may be quite strong. Including a variety of physical activities may be helpful in preventing boredom, and including some element of socialization, such as exercising with friends or family members, can help, too.

7. SURVIVORSHIP CARE PLANS

A survivorship care plan is a document that contains information about the kind of cancer the survivor had, as well as the type and duration of treatment. In addition, it might contain information about the kinds of tests the survivor needs to have in the future. Many survivors don't know the details of their cancer or treatment, but this is important information to have on hand.

There are many different survivorship care plans available. Some are intended to be completed by the health care team and then shared with the survivor's primary care provider as well as the survivor. Others can be completed online by the survivor, assuming that he or she knows the details of the cancer diagnosis and treatment.

Although the contents of these care plans differ, they usually contain the following information: the kind of cancer, including stage and grade; a summary of the treatment, including surgery, chemotherapy, radiation, and adjuvant treatment (the amount and dose of drugs and radiation are usually provided); the schedule for follow-up blood tests, X-rays, CT scans, and MRI tests; the schedule for follow-up medical appointments with an appropriate provider (a specialist versus a primary care provider); information about risks to the patient and how to identify signs of recurrence; information about long-term side effects of treatment; recommendations for healthy lifestyle practices, including diet and exercise, smoking cessation, and risk modification; and other resources for the survivor and his or her family. The survivorship care plan is often presented in paper format but may also be available online. The contents of the survivorship care plan are usually discussed by the oncology care team with the patient (and parents, when appropriate) to ensure that he or she understands the information and has an opportunity to ask questions.

The Institute of Medicine published a report in 2005 titled "From Cancer Patient to Cancer Survivor: Lost in Transition," which has become the definitive guide for survivorship care in North America. This landmark report recognizes survivorship as a distinct phase of the cancer journey, and one that needs to be recognized as such by cancer specialists and other health care providers. A key aspect of providing care for cancer survivors is ensuring that all members of the patient's care team, including the patient and family, know what is expected after primary treatment ends. Knowing what has been done, what needs to be done in the future, and by whom is found to be as important as the details of the recommended plan.

8. FERTILITY ISSUES

Many treatments for cancer have the potential to negatively affect fertility. Chemotherapy is the most likely culprit; however, radiation therapy to the pelvic area and surgery also have the potential to affect fertility in cancer survivors. Dealing with infertility can be very frustrating and a source of distress for most couples who experience it. Couples faced with infertility have levels of depression twice those of the normal population. Emotional well-being, relationship satisfaction, and sexuality are also compromised.

The impact of chemotherapy on future fertility should be discussed with every patient of childbearing age, and it should also be discussed with the parents of children diagnosed with cancer. But in the crisis of the moment, the topic may not be addressed. For one thing, the newly diagnosed person may not want to talk about it. When your life is threatened by cancer, you may not consider future fertility to be as important. For the parents of a young child with cancer, this may be the furthest thing from their minds as they face the potential loss of their precious child. For another thing, the health care provider may decide that fertility is not an important topic to be discussed. This is a paternalistic attitude, but it does exist. Finally, the discussion may be initiated in a very superficial way or the patient may not be able to take it all in, given the large amount of information to be absorbed in such a short time frame.

In a nationwide study of oncologists, 30 percent said that they rarely consider a woman patient's desire for fertility when planning treatment. Their focus is on curing the cancer. Less than half of the oncologists in another study routinely referred their female cancer patients to a specialist in fertility preservation. Other studies have found that between one- and two-thirds of women with cancer are not told about the effects of treatment on fertility, and those who are told want even more information than they are given.

Infertility is known to cause significant conflict for many couples. Even though no cause may be found for the infertility, the couple may blame each other. There are also significant costs associated with the diagnosis and treatment of infertility, which can put additional strain on the partnership. One partner may be more interested in having children than the other, and this can also cause conflict.

Many couples try to find information on the Internet, and although there is a lot of information out there, not all of it is useful or valid. Anyone can set up a website, and many people do just that, with their personal experience published for all to see. Their opinions are not necessarily reliable or valid and are merely personal expressions. Stories on the Web can be very touching, but they can also be upsetting. Websites that look like legitimate sources of information may be the window dressing of a for-profit agency that wants to hook you in and take your money, with no regard for integrity. If it sounds too good to be true (e.g., "99 percent of our patients conceive in the first month"), then it likely is.

For women whose fertility may be negatively affected by cancer treatment, deciding what to do can be very difficult. Complex decisions have to be made in a time of crisis. Fertility-preserving options have to be weighed against life-saving treatment. And the options for fertility preservation for women are limited. The best option for a woman with cancer whose treatment may affect her fertility is to harvest her eggs and create embryos with her partner's sperm. The embryos are then frozen for implantation at a future time. This method is the most successful (with a greater than 50 percent chance of success), but there are drawbacks. Treatment for the cancer has to be delayed for at least one menstrual cycle, and the woman has to take medication to stimulate the ovaries to produce multiple eggs. This is done with hormones, and women with hormone-dependent cancers usually should not be exposed to additional hormones. It is also dependent on having a partner who can donate sperm for fertilization.

There are other potential strategies for preserving fertility in women, but these remain experimental, with very low levels of success. These include freezing eggs (with a less than 4 percent chance of success) and freezing ovarian tissue that is put back into the woman after treatment is complete (still experimental due to very limited success so far).

For women who need pelvic radiation as treatment, it is common practice to shield the ovaries from the field of radiation or even to move them surgically out of the radiation field. Radiation to the pelvis may result in anatomical changes to the uterus, so even if the woman is able to become pregnant, the chances of a successful outcome are limited by the ability of the uterus itself to hold a pregnancy.

The best option for fertility preservation is for men with cancer. Freezing sperm for later use is a highly successful and well-established practice. However, the man must know about this option *before* treatment starts and must have enough time to donate sperm samples (usually two or three times, forty-eight hours apart) and have them frozen. In the rush to begin treatment, this does not always happen, and an opportunity is lost. For young men and boys, the reality of one day having children just may not be something that they consider important, and so it is not done.

Care should be taken when choosing a fertility clinic or doctor. It really is "buyer beware" because not all clinics are run by credible doctors. Treating infertility is a business for some, and people desperate to have children can be cheated by false promises and statistics. It is important to check the credentials of the doctors at any clinic by seeing if they are associated with the American Society of Reproductive Medicine (www.asrm.org) or with an academic teaching hospital. This will in part help to ensure that the doctors associated with the clinic are well qualified.

9. COGNITIVE DIFFICULTIES

Cancer- or cancer-treatment-associated cognitive change is a well-described phenomenon sometimes called "chemo-brain." Changes in cognition can occur at any point in the cancer journey, and many people report changes to their cognitive functioning as a result of treatment for cancer.

Cancer-related cognitive changes can present themselves in different ways. Some people may have difficulty concentrating, staying focused, or paying attention. Visual memory can also be affected. These signs can be quite subtle and may be attributed to other causes, such as poor sleep, fatigue, or just making a mistake. However, when there is a pattern or these signs are consistent, it is likely due to something other than coincidence.

Poor-quality sleep or sleep that is disturbed can play a role in one's ability to cope and be efficient during the day. Hot flashes at night are sometimes called night sweats because they cause excessive sweating that wakes the person up. They are often associated with menopause and can be particularly bad for women who have been put into menopause by chemotherapy. They often are also very bad for women who take antiestrogen medication as part of their treatment for breast cancer. A lack of estrogen in a woman's body is known to cause hot flashes and can be extremely bothersome. Organizational skills and executive functioning can also be affected after cancer treatment. Any alteration in one's ability to function normally can be both frustrating and frightening, but when it involves work-related issues, it can be very serious indeed.

Cognitive functioning may also be affected by cancer and its treatment in other ways: verbal memory (remembering words or things that have been read), motor functioning (using your hands to complete a task or misjudging the edge of a coffee table and dropping a cup), information processing (getting confused about what is being said to you), and language ability (having difficulty finding the right words).

Accepting that this is happening can be very challenging. We often have little insight into our own functioning, or we may be actively in denial about what is really going on. And often family members are reluctant to bring up problems for fear of upsetting someone they love. It is also often difficult to accept that things are not as they used to be or should be. People often find ways to compensate for forgetfulness, or the signs are so subtle that everyone around you makes allowances.

There are a number of tests available to identify specific areas where cognition is altered. But the tests are not very accurate, and the results can be difficult to interpret. Unfortunately, knowing the area affected does not provide clear interventions for treatment, either. It is suggested that listening to the patient's reported symptoms rather than relying on tests is the best way to go, based on the present level of knowledge in this area.

There is some evidence that a psychostimulant called methylphenidate is useful in the treatment of cancer-related cognitive changes. This medication is commonly used to treat attention-deficit hyperactivity disorder. Like any other medication, it can have significant side effects, but studies in women with cancer have shown benefits.

It has also been suggested that because cognitive changes are so common after treatment for cancer, the risk for this should be part of the consent process before someone starts treatment. This approach has not gained significant support, so patients are often not warned that cognitive changes may occur.

There has been a lot of research on helping the elderly with cognitive decline, and many of these strategies can be helpful for the person with cancer-related cognitive changes. Merely knowing that the changes are due to the cancer or its treatment can be reassuring. People often think they are going crazy, and reassurance can help them start adapting to the changes.

These changes are not related to other neurological conditions that are progressive (such as Alzheimer's disease) and do not indicate any change in the recovery from cancer. They are also not related to the recurrence of cancer. Strategies for coping with these challenges include using written reminders of tasks to be accomplished, employing an electronic device such as a digital diary to send audible alerts when tasks have to be performed, and keeping a detailed calendar of events with sticky notes that can be removed and carried to act as reminders.

Exercise has been shown to help as well. It improves strength and stamina and promotes oxygenation of the brain. Reducing or eliminating background noise and limiting concurrent multiple tasks can also help concentration. Doing intellectually stimulating activities such as crossword puzzles and sudoku can help exercise the brain and has been shown to maintain brain activity in the elderly.

Making lists is a useful way of identifying what needs to be done. It also helps to break down what may seem to be a complex set of actions into smaller, more manageable steps. Many people use lists for all sorts of things: to be reminded of what they have to do, to weigh the pros and cons of a certain action, and to help them focus on details.

· 12 ·

Resources

This chapter provides the reader with a comprehensive list of print and Web resources for successful living after cancer. It also highlights educational programs and professional resources supporting cancer survivors.

PROGRESSIVE RELAXATION

In chapter 2, the social worker recommends that Nancy, a young woman with breast cancer, try progressive relaxation as a strategy to help reduce her fear and anxiety related to recurrence. This is a simple technique that can be done just before bed, anytime during the day when you have fifteen minutes to yourself, or when you feel anxious and out of control. It is easy to learn and does not require special equipment. It reduces physical tension in the muscles of the body and promotes mental relaxation.

An important aspect of this is to concentrate on the feelings or sensations you experience when your muscles are first tense and then relaxed. With practice, you will be able to relax your body without first tensing your muscles so that when you feel muscle tension, you can just tell your body to relax, and it will.

To start, you should sit in a comfortable chair and breathe deeply for a few minutes. Then, starting with your feet and lower legs, tense the muscles of your feet and calves by flexing your feet and tightening the muscles of your calves and legs. Hold this for five seconds and think about how it feels. Then exhale as you relax those muscles and consciously think about how the relaxed muscles feel. Then contract the muscles of your thighs by straightening your knees and squeezing your legs together. Hold for five seconds and then relax

189

as you breathe out. Remember the sensations in your muscles when they are first contracted and then relaxed. Continue to breathe with slow, deep, regular breaths using your abdominal muscles to pull air into your lungs.

Continue up your body toward your head. You will need to contract and relax the muscles moving up—from your legs to your buttocks and abdomen, your upper back, your arms, your chin, your neck and shoulders, and finally your jaw and facial muscles. Once you have reached your head, allow a feeling of relaxation to flow down your body as you continue to breathe deeply and slowly. Remember the feeling of relaxation so that you can return to it when you need or want to. It gets easier and easier with practice.

For optimal results, you should practice this relaxation exercise at least three times a week for fifteen minutes at a time. Eventually you will be able to feel relaxed just by thinking about being relaxed! It may be helpful to keep a score card of your level of tension before and after each session—write down the date and time and your level of tension before you start (from 0 = no tension to 10 = the worst tension you have felt) and then again afterward and chart your progress over the days of practice.

DEEP BREATHING

Don't we all know how to breathe? After all, we've been doing it since the moment we entered this world. But many of us don't breathe deeply and properly. Close your eyes for a moment and breathe as you normally do. Take note of how your chest moves as you inhale and exhale. Most of us breathe just in the upper part of our lungs—our breaths are shallow, and only our chests rise and fall. We don't take in enough oxygen with each breath, and it can actually trigger anxiety for some of us. This type of breathing is similar to the rapid breathing that occurs during situations of high anxiety. Imagine being chased by a lion and how you would breathe—shallow, rapid breaths with tense muscles in the chest, shoulder, and neck.

A much healthier way to breathe is to involve the abdominal muscles with each inhalation and exhalation. Put your hand on your stomach and feel how it moves when you take in a deep, slow breath and let it out the same way. You should always breathe that way, and it helps to keep you relaxed. Practice this when you do your progressive muscle relaxation exercises and remind yourself during your usual daily activities to breathe with your stomach muscles. When belly breathing becomes the way you normally breathe, you will notice that you feel more relaxed as you go about your daily activities.

MINDFULNESS MEDITATION AND STRESS REDUCTION

Mindfulness practice is a way of being in the moment, fully aware of what is going on around us. It is based on an ancient Buddhist philosophy and spirituality but is nondenominational and nonreligious. It has been used successfully in the management of many different kinds of medical and psychiatric conditions, including pain disorders, depression, anxiety, substance abuse, eating disorders, fibromyalgia, and child behavior problems.

Mindfulness-based stress reduction is an intervention that was pioneered by Dr. Jon Kabat Zinn almost thirty years ago and has been offered at the University of Massachusetts and other health care facilities as a formal program for many years. Dr. Kabat Zinn has written a number of books for the general public and has produced a number of CDs that support the learning and practice of mindfulness meditation.

Mindfulness has been used for people with cancer across the illness experience, from diagnosis through survival. It has been shown to help reduce distress, to promote coping and relaxation, and to alleviate both physical and mental pain. Mindfulness is particularly helpful when someone feels out of control and helpless, a common experience during cancer treatment. Mindfulness helps to manage that out-of-control feeling by drawing the person toward an inward locus of control and consciously directing thoughts to the present moment instead of to an uncertain future or an unhappy memory of events in the past.

There are four forms of mindfulness practice: awareness of sensations, sitting meditation, body scan, and mindful movement. In awareness of sensations, patients are taught to focus their complete attention on different sensory experiences such as sounds or tastes or sights. One way to do this is to focus on the sensation of breathing while sitting quietly and comfortably with your eyes closed. As described in the section on deep breathing, this elicits a sensation of total relaxation, and individuals can return to this deep breathing when they feel stressed or anxious. The breath itself becomes a safe place to retreat to when uncertainty challenges them and they become anxious or afraid.

The next step is to become aware of the body and its sensations during sitting meditation. When you focus your attention on a physical sensation, it actually helps to control that sensation. For example, focusing on the sensation of pain in the moment blocks the negative thoughts associated with the pain itself (Why am I having this pain? When will it go away? What does it mean? Is my cancer getting worse?). It will also draw attention to the nature of the pain and how it ebbs and flows, showing us that it is not constant and that it is not completely overwhelming. The same can be experienced with feelings and emotions. Fear also ebbs and flows when you focus solely on what the fear feels like and not on the many thoughts that flow from it.

Mindfulness interventions have been studied in people with different kinds of cancer (breast, prostate, gynecological) and have shown positive effects on distress and anxiety as well as on negative coping mechanisms.

The body scan is the third form of mindfulness meditation, and in some ways it is similar to progressive relaxation in that you focus awareness on the body, but this time moving from your head to your feet. Deliberately focusing on how each part of your body is feeling can reconnect us with our body in a kind and loving manner. It can also help one get in touch with what one's body really needs in the moment—warmth, perhaps, or food, or deliberate relaxation of tense muscles. Finally, mindful movement, such as with a form of yoga, can help us get in touch with our body in movement and its strengths and flexibility.

One way of exploring mindfulness is to think about some of the things we do in our daily lives. What happened to you in the shower or bath this morning? Did you stand or lie under the warm water, experiencing the sensation of the water as it flowed over and around your body? Did you smell the fragrance of the soap or shampoo as your fingers moved through your hair and over your scalp? Did you really feel the softness of the towel as you moved it over your body and your skin emerged, dry and soft and clean?

Most of us hurry through this daily experience, thinking about what lies ahead for us during the busyness of our day. We don't feel the water, smell the shampoo, or appreciate the texture of the towel. We are not *in the moment* but rather somewhere else, already feeling the stress of what we have to do, the traffic we will have to negotiate, or the meeting we will have to attend. Our emotions follow along, and we are stressed and exhausted before we even start the day. By being mindful, by truly being in the moment, we can enhance the experience of what it is we are doing.

People with cancer are often very focused on the past and the future—memories of painful events and fear of the future can overwhelm and prevent the person from being fully alive in the moment without the pain of the past or the fear of the unknown. Mindfulness helps bring the focus to the present, and even if there is fear or pain in the present moment, being fully attentive to it, without clouding it with memories and the unknown of the future, can help the person cope with the immediate emotions and sensations.

Here are some useful resources for learning about mindfulness:

Letting Everything Become Your Teacher: 100 Lessons in Mindfulness, by Jon Kabat Zinn (2009). Delta Publishing.
Arriving at Your Own Door: 108 Lessons in Mindfulness, by Jon Kabat Zinn (2007). Hyperion Books.

Mindfulness for Beginners, by Jon Kabat Zinn (CD, 2006). Sounds True, Inc.
Coming to Our Senses: Healing Ourselves and the World through Mindfulness, by Jon Kabat Zinn (2006). Hyperion Books.
Wherever You Go, There You Are, by Jon Kabat Zinn (2005). Hyperion Books.
Full Catastrophe Living: Using the Wisdom of Your Body and Mind to Face Stress, Pain, and Illness, by Jon Kabat Zinn (1990). Delta Publishing.
Guided Mindfulness Meditation, by Jon Kabat Zinn (CD, 2005). Sounds True, Inc.

SENSUAL MASSAGE AND SENSATE FOCUS-EXERCISES

One of the most useful couple-oriented activities for enhancing mutual sexual enjoyment is a series of touching exercises called sensate focus. Masters and Johnson labeled this technique and have used it as a basic step in treating sexual problems. It can be helpful in reducing anxiety caused by goal orientation and for increasing communication, pleasure, and closeness. This technique is by no means appropriate only for sex therapy but can be used by all couples to enhance their sexual relationships. In the sensate-focus touching exercises, partners take turns touching each other while following some essential guidelines. Of course, homosexual as well as heterosexual couples can do these exercises.

Sensual Message

Establish ground rules, which might include the following:

- Determine who will be the first giver.
- Establish whether you and your partner will be clothed or unclothed.
- Choose a location where you both will be comfortable, preferably not the bed.
- Dim the lights and play soft music you both enjoy.
- Use plenty of pillows or a comforter.
- If you wish, use baby oils, scented oils, lotions, or powder.
- Tell the giver what feels good and what does not.
- Sensual massage omits the genitals and breasts, which are discussed in the sensate-focus section.
- Begin with facial caressing. Normally the giver sits and the receiver lies flat on his or her back with the head resting on the giver's thighs. With the hands well lubricated, the giver begins with the chin, then

strokes the cheeks, forehead, and temples. Caress the face as if you were a blind person seeking a mental picture of your partner. Then explore the ear lobes, lips, and the nose before returning to massage the temples for complete relaxation. Rest, talk about the experience, and reverse roles again.

- Massage the remainder of the body tenderly, and be attentive to your feelings. Then reverse roles again.

Goals of the touching exercise include the following:

- to show dedication toward enriching the relationship,
- to express needs and desires in new ways,
- to find out how each partner likes to touch and be touched,
- to explore new patterns of pleasuring that do not always have to be sexual,
- to help the relationship grow, and
- to reduce the fear of physical changes of aging.

Sensate-Focus Exercises

Sensate-focus exercises were introduced by researchers Masters and Johnson to treat couples with sexual problems. The exercises offer an approach to sexual enrichment. The exercises are divided into four progressive stages. Master each stage before moving to the next. Repeat all previous stages each time. The pace depends on your progress and comfort.

Here are some helpful suggestions:

- The toucher learns from the one being touched. The one being touched takes the partner's hand and thus controls the degree of pressure as well as the pattern and length of strokes. This is a learning experience for the giver as well as the receiver.
- The learning hand of the toucher should not be his or her dominant hand. A right-handed person should use the left hand, and left-handers, the right hand.
- Do the exercises when you and your partner are rested and not pressed for time. Don't do the exercises after a heavy meal or when you have had a disagreement.
- Do the exercises early in the morning when male testosterone levels are higher.
- At no time is there to be any attempt to have sexual intercourse, even if it is the man's first erection in months.

- After the session, discuss what you think you have accomplished and share positive as well as negative feelings with your partner.

Stages of Sensate Focus

The partners take turns being the giver and the receiver. Communication during the exercises is done by guiding the hand of the partner giving the massage. Limit talking until after the exercises are completed.

First stage: Limit touching and stroking to the areas of the body that are not sexually stimulating.

Second stage: Touch, stroke, and explore the sensual responses of the entire body, including the breasts and genitals, without the intent of bringing about erection or vaginal lubrication. At this stage, some talk may be helpful.

Third stage: Repeat the first two stages. Stroke the penis and clitoris and probe the vaginal opening with the finger. Note erectile and lubricative responses.

Fourth stage: Repeat the first three stages. Caress and stimulate breasts and genitals. Use a lubricant, especially for the clitoris, the outer lips, and the vaginal opening of the pre- and postmenopausal woman, as well as for the male with less than full erectile response. When the man's erection is firm enough to attempt penetration, the couple will want to insert the penis and feel it in the vagina.

If the female feels that her partner is losing his erection, she can initiate pelvic movements until it returns. Containment can produce anxiety for some men. However, there is no demand for either partner to perform. The exercise continues as long as the couple feels comfortable with one another and are enjoying and savoring the good feelings.

The use of baby oil or body lotion is recommended for stages one and two of the sensate-focus exercises. A sexual lubricant is helpful during stages three and four when the genitals are touched.

LUBRICANTS AND MOISTURIZERS

Lubricants are products designed to make vaginal penetration more comfortable. They can be used for sexual activity and also when you have to use a dilator after radiation therapy. There are a number of these available at the drugstore or supermarket, and most are water based.

The most well known of the lubricants is K-Y Jelly, which is used just before sexual activity. It tends to dry out quite quickly during intercourse and gets sticky. A more effective alternative is a lubricant called Astroglide. This glycerin-based product does not get sticky even after prolonged use and can be replenished with water if it does start to dry out. Some women find that the glycerin may cause vaginal yeast infections. There is now a version of Astroglide that is glycerin free. Both of these products are now available in a warming variety, which can add some spice to sex play, but care should be taken if the sensitive vaginal tissues are irritated, as the warming ingredient can make this worse. There are also some other water-based lubricants that do not contain glycerin. Examples include Liquid Silk, Slippery Stuff, Oh My, Sensual Organics, and Probe. These are usually found only online or in sex stores.

Silicone lubricants (such as K-Y Intrigue, Eros, and Wet Platinum) stay fluid much longer and are not absorbed by the skin. They are safe to use for sex play and intercourse and are not associated with the kind of silicone used in breast implants. They are *very* slippery, and any residue left behind needs to be cleaned off with soap and water. The silicone can also be slippery on wet bathroom surfaces. These lubricants cause deterioration of silicone dilators or sex toys and so should not be used with these. Silicone lubricants may be more difficult to find in drugstores but can be found in sex stores or online (www.blowfish.com). However, K-Y Intrigue is available in most drugstores.

Oil-based lubricants such as petroleum jelly are generally not recommended for vaginal intercourse. They destroy latex condoms and can be irritating to the tissues of the vulva. However, they are good for male masturbation. Some women use olive oil, coconut oil, vitamin E oil, or cocoa butter because they are more natural. Generally, anything that you can eat can be used in the vagina or on the vulva. They do stain sheets, but they are inexpensive and easily available. Clear mineral oil may be used as well, but these often contain petroleum and should be used with caution (check the label!).

Moisturizers are intended to provide additional moisture to the vagina and are not intended to be used during sexual activity. Two of the most well known and easily available brands are Replens and K-Y Liquibeads.

Replens is a clear gel that is inserted into the vagina three times a week using a plastic applicator. It works by drawing moisture into the walls of the vagina. Initially women report an increased amount of vaginal discharge that they may find distasteful, but this usually resolves after a few weeks. Many women find that they are able to use Replens less often than the recommended three times a week once more comfortable levels of vaginal moisture are achieved.

Liquibeads are round ovules containing a mixture of silicone and glycerin encased in a gelatin coating. They are inserted into the vagina with a special applicator every three to four days, where they dissolve and coat the vaginal walls. Because they contain silicone, they likely serve a dual purpose as a lubricant as well.

Some women find that vitamin E oil is also an effective moisturizer. The oil usually comes in a small capsule that can be punctured with a pin. The oil is then placed on a finger and gently rubbed on the vulva and inside the vagina. It is much cheaper than either Replens or Liquibeads.

SURVIVORSHIP CARE PLANS

In chapter 8, you learned about survivorship care plans and their important role for cancer survivors after treatment is over. Some cancer centers and hospitals have these care plans and share them with the cancer survivor and family, as well as with the family physician or other primary care provider. Other hospitals do not routinely offer these to patients. You can ask if your oncology care team provides these documents, and if not, you may complete one yourself with their help. Here is a list of websites that provide templates or guidelines for care plans.

Journey Forward (www.journeyforward.org)
This website provides a template for a survivorship care plan that is filled out by your oncology team and then shared with you and your primary care provider.

National Comprehensive Cancer Network (www.nccn.org)
This website provides evidence-based information and guidelines for your health care providers.

LIVESTRONG care plan (www.livestrongcareplan.org)
The team from LIVESTRONG and the Lance Armstrong Foundation provides an opportunity to create your own survivorship care plan.

Prescription for Living (www.tiny.cc/SFA8e)
This is another template for a survivorship care plan that can be completed by your oncology care team.

Cure Search Children's Oncology Group (www.survivorshipguidelines.org)
This website provides guidelines for follow-up care for children and teenagers with cancer.

FERTILITY ORGANIZATIONS

In chapter 9, you read about a couple facing the challenges of not being able to have a baby after cancer treatment. Finding help for this can be difficult. There are many fertility clinics across North America, but how do you find one that can help after cancer? How do you know that you will not be given false hopes and promises while you spend many months and many dollars trying to get pregnant? Here is a list of reputable websites and services that may be able to help.

The American Society for Reproductive Medicine (www.asrm.org)
The American Society for Reproductive Medicine is a nonprofit organization whose members must demonstrate the high ethical principles of the medical profession; show an interest in infertility, reproductive medicine, and biology; and adhere to the objectives of the organization. The website contains information specifically for people with cancer.

The American Fertility Association (www.theafa.org)
The American Fertility Association is a national nonprofit organization that provides services and materials free of charge to consumers, including an extensive online library, monthly online "webinars," telephone and in-person coaching, a resource directory, an "ask the experts" online feature, daily fertility news, and a toll-free support line.

Fertile Hope (www.fertilehope.org)
Fertile Hope is a national LIVESTRONG initiative dedicated to providing reproductive information, support, and hope to cancer patients and survivors whose medical treatments present the risk of infertility.

WEBSITES

Where can you find more information about cancer survivorship? Here are some reputable organizations and their websites:

> Centers for Disease Control: www.cdc.gov/cancer/survivorship
> National Cancer Institute, Office of Cancer Survivorship: http://dccps.nci
> .nih.gov/ocs
> National Coalition for Cancer Survivorship: www.canceradvocacy.org
> CancerCare: www.cancercare.org

American Cancer Society: www.cancer.org
Patient Advocate Foundation: www.patientadvocate.org
LIVESTRONG (formerly the Lance Armstrong Foundation): www
.livestrong.org

BOOKS

The Cancer Survivor's Guide: The Essential Handbook to Life after Cancer, by Michael Feuerstein MPH and Patricia Findley. Da Capo Press, 2006.
Picking Up the Pieces: Moving Forward after Surviving Cancer, by Sherri Magee and Kathy Scalzo. Rutgers University Press, 2007.
After Cancer: A Guide to Your New Life, by Wendy S. Harpham. Harper Paperbacks, 1995.
Everyone's Guide to Cancer Survivorship: A Road Map for Better Health, by Ernest Rosenbaum, David Spiegel, Patricia Fobair, and Holly Gautier. Andrews McMeel, 2007.
Handbook of Cancer Survivorship, by Michael Feuerstein. Springer, 2007.
From Cancer Patient to Cancer Survivor: Lost in Transition, by the Institute of Medicine and the National Research Council of the National Academies. National Academy of Sciences, 2006.
Crazy Sex Cancer Survivor, by Kris Carr. The Globe Pequot Press, 2008.
Everything Changes: The Insider's Guide to Cancer in your 20s and 30s, by Kairol Rosenthal. John Wiley and Sons, 2009.
100 Questions and Answers about Life after Cancer: A Survivor's Guide, by Page Tolbert and Penny Damaskos. Jones and Bartlett, 2008.
What Helped Me Get Through: Cancer Survivors Share Wisdom and Hope, edited by Julie Silver. American Cancer Society, 2009.

Bibliography

CHAPTER 2: IS THE CANCER BACK?

Armes, Jo, Maggie Crowe, et al. "Patients' supportive care needs beyond the end of cancer treatment: A prospective, longitudinal survey." *Journal of Clinical Oncology* 27 (2009): 6172–79.

Gil, Karen, Merle Mishel, et al. "Triggers of uncertainty about recurrence and long-term treatment side effects in older African American and Caucasian breast cancer survivors." *Oncology Nursing Forum* 31 (2004): 633–39.

Mehnert, Anja, Petra Berg, et al. "Fear of cancer progression and cancer-related intrusive cognitions in breast cancer survivors." *Psycho-Oncology* 18 (2009): 1273–80.

Mellon, Suzanne, Trace Kershaw, et al. "A family-based model to predict fear of recurrence for cancer survivors and their care givers." *Psycho-Oncology* 16 (2007): 214–23.

Thong, Melissa, Floortje Mols, et al. "The impact of disease progression on perceived health status and quality of life of long-term cancer survivors." *Journal of Cancer Survivorship* 3 (2009): 164–73.

Vivar, Christina, Navidad Canga, et al. "The psychosocial impact of recurrence on cancer survivors and family members: A narrative review." *Journal of Advanced Nursing* 65 (2009): 724–36.

CHAPTER 3: WHEN WILL I BE HAPPY AGAIN?

Fulcher, Caryl, Terry Badger, et al. "Putting evidence into practice: Interventions for depression." *Clinical Journal of Oncology Nursing* 12 (2008): 131–40.

Hamer, Mark, Yoichi Chida, and Gerard Molloy. "Psychological distress and cancer mortality." *Journal of Psychosomatic Research* 66 (2009): 255–58.

Pirl, William, Joseph Greer, et al. "Major depressive disorder in long-term cancer survivors: Analysis of the National Comorbidity Survey replication." *Journal of Clinical Oncology* 27 (2009): 4130–34.

Rabin, Elaine, Elizeth Heldt, et al. "Depression and perceptions of quality of life of breast cancer survivors and their male partners." *Oncology Nursing Forum* 36 (2009): E153–E158.

Rancour, Patrice. "Using archetypes and transitions theory to help patients move from active treatment to survivorship." *Clinical Journal of Oncology Nursing* 12 (2009): 935–40.

Reich, Michael. "Depression and cancer: Recent data on clinical issues, research challenges and treatment approaches." *Current Opinions in Oncology* 20 (2008): 353–59.

CHAPTER 4: WHAT WILL EVERYONE SAY?

De Boer, Angela, Taina Taskila, et al. "Cancer survivors and unemployment: A meta-analysis and meta-regression." *Journal of the American Medical Association* 301 (2009): 753–62.

Hoving, J. L., and M. L. A. Broekhuizen. "Return to work of breast cancer survivors: A systematic review of intervention studies." *BMC Cancer* 9 (2009): 117–27.

Mols, Floortje, Melissa Thong, et al. "Long-term cancer survivors experience work changes after diagnosis: Results of a population-based study." *Psycho-Oncology* 18 (2009): 1252–60.

CHAPTER 5: WHY DO I FEEL SO TIRED?

Barsevick, Andrea, Tracey Newhall, and Susan Brown. "Management of cancer-related fatigue." *Clinical Journal of Oncology Nursing* 12 (2008): 21–25.

Breitbart, William, and Yesne Alici. "Pharmacologic treatment options for cancer-related fatigue: Current state of clinical research." *Clinical Journal of Oncology Nursing* 12 (2008): 27–36.

Cheville, Andrea. "Cancer-related fatigue." *Physical Medicine Rehabilitation Clinics of North America* 20 (2009): 405–16.

Kangas, Maria, Dana Bovbjerg, and Guy Montgomery. "Cancer-related fatigue: A systematic and meta-analysis review of non-pharmacological therapies for cancer patients." *Psychological Bulletin* 134 (2008): 700–41.

Kuchinski, Anne-Marie, Maria Reading, and Ayham Lash. "Treatment-related fatigue and exercise in patients with cancer: A systematic review." *MEDSURG Nursing* 18 (2009): 174–80.

Schwartz, Anne. "Fatigue in long-term cancer survivors." *Oncology Nurse Edition* 23 (2009): 1–4.

CHAPTER 6: WHERE DID THAT FEELING GO?

Horeden, Amanda, and Annette Street. "Issues of intimacy and sexuality in the face of cancer: The patient perspective." *Cancer Nursing* 30 (2007): E11–E18.

Katz, Anne. *Breaking the Silence on Cancer and Sexuality: A Handbook for Healthcare Providers*. Pittsburgh: Oncology Nursing Society, 2007.

Katz, Anne. *Woman Cancer Sex*. Pittsburgh: Hygeia Media, 2009.

Schover, Leslie. "Sexuality and fertility after cancer." *Hematology* (2005): 523–27.

CHAPTER 7: FEELING FIT

Bellizzi, Keith, Julia Rowland, et al. "Health behaviors of cancer survivors: Examining opportunities for cancer control intervention." *Journal of Clinical Oncology* 23 (2005): 8884–93.

Blanchard, Christopher, Kerry Courneya, and Kevin Stein. "Cancer survivors' adherence to lifestyle behavior recommendations and associations with health-related quality of life: Results from the American Cancer Society's SCS-II." *Journal of Clinical Oncology* 26 (2008): 2198–2204.

Findley, Patricia, and Usha Sambamoorthi. "Preventive health services and lifestyle practices in cancer survivors: A population health investigation." *Journal of Cancer Survivorship* 3 (2009): 43–58.

Irwin, Melinda, and Susan Mayne. "Impact of nutrition and exercise on cancer survival." *The Cancer Journal* 14 (2008): 435–41.

Mosher, Catherine, Richard Sloane, et al. "Associations between lifestyle factors and quality of life among older, long-term breast, prostate, and colorectal cancer survivors." *Cancer* 115 (2009): 4001–9.

Rabin, Carolyn, and Bernardine Pinto. "Cancer-related beliefs and health behavior change among breast cancer survivors and their first-degree relatives." *Psycho-Oncology* 15 (2006): 701–12.

Schmitz, Kathryn, Kerry Courneya, et al. "American College of Sports Medicine roundtable on exercise guidelines for cancer survivors." *Medicine & Science in Sports & Exercise* (2010): 1409–26.

CHAPTER 8: WHAT SHOULD I BE LOOKING FOR?

Cantrell, Mary Ann, and Teresa Conte. "Between being cured and being healed: The paradox of childhood cancer survivorship." *Qualitative Health Research* 19 (2009): 312–22.

Earle, Craig. "Failing to plan is planning to fail: Improving the quality of care with survivorship care plans." *Journal of Clinical Oncology* 32 (2006): 5112–16.

Haylock, Pamela, Sandra Mitchell, et al. "The cancer survivor's prescription for living." *American Journal of Nursing* 107 (2007): 58–69.

Hoffman, Barbara, and Ellen Stovall. "Survivorship perspectives and advocacy." *Journal of Clinical Oncology* 32 (2006): 5154–59.

Houlihan, Nancy. "Transitioning to cancer survivorship: Plans of care." *Oncology Nurse Edition* 23 (2009): 1–7.

Michel, G., D. M. Greenfield, et al. "Follow-up care after childhood cancer: Survivors' expectations and preferences for care." *European Journal of Cancer* 45 (2009): 1616–23.

CHAPTER 9: WE WANT TO START A FAMILY

Chang, Hye Jin, and Chang Suk Suh. "Fertility preservation for women with malignancies: Current developments of cryopreservation." *Journal of Gynecological Oncology* 19 (2008): 99–107.

Duffy, Christine, and Susan Allen. "Medical and psychosocial aspects of fertility after cancer." *Cancer Journal* 15 (2009): 27–33.

Hobbie, Wendy, Suan Ogle, and Jill Ginsberg. "Fertility concerns for young males undergoing cancer therapy." *Seminars in Oncology Nursing* 25 (2009): 245–50.

Nagel, Kim, Jane Cassano, et al. "Collaborative multidisciplinary team approach to fertility issues among adolescent and young adult cancer patients." *International Journal of Nursing Practice* 15 (2009): 311–17.

Nagel, Kim, and Michael Neal. "Discussions regarding sperm banking with adolescent and young adult males who have cancer." *Journal of Pediatric Oncology Nursing* 25 (2008): 102–6.

Olsthoorn-Heim, Els, and Guido de Wert. "Ovarian tissue cryopreservation: Promises and uncertainties." *European Journal of Health Law* 16 (2009): 173–83.

Schover, Leslie. "Patient attitudes toward fertility preservation." *Pediatric Blood Cancer* 53 (2009): 281–84.

Tschudin, Sibil, and Johannes Bitzer. "Psychological aspects of fertility preservation in men and women affected by cancer and other life-threatening diseases." *Human Reproduction Update* 15 (2009): 587–97.

CHAPTER 10: AM I LOSING MY MIND?

Dietrich, Jorg, and Michelle Monje. "Clinical patterns and biological correlates of cognitive dysfunction associated with cancer therapy." *The Oncologist* 13 (2008): 1285–95.

Hurria, Arti, George Somio, and Tim Ahles. "Renaming 'Chemobrain.'" *Cancer Investigations* 25 (2007): 373–77.

Nail, Lillian. "Cognitive changes in cancer survivors." *American Journal of Nursing* 106 (2006): 48–54.

Nelson, Christian, Nina Nandy, and Andrew Roth. "Chemotherapy and cognitive deficits: Mechanisms, findings, and potential interventions." *Palliative and Supportive Care* 5 (2007): 273–80.

Staat, Kari, and Milena Segatore. "The phenomenon of chemo brain." *Clinical Journal of Oncology Nursing* 9 (2005): 713–21.

Index

American Association of Sex Educators, Counselors and Therapists (AASECT), 97
Americans with Disabilities Act (ADA), 52, 56
antidepressant, 41–42
antiestrogen, 152, 156, 162

back to work plan, 60, 167
bladder cancer, 105–106
breast cancer, 10, 151;
  treatment of, 10

chemotherapy, 153
chemo-brain, 153, 162
childbearing, 9, 183–85
childhood cancer, 120, 122, 125, 136
cognitive behaviorial therapy, 42, 44
cognitive changes, 9;
  symptoms of, 155, 158;
  testing for, 162;
  treatment of, 162–63, 166, 186–87
colon cancer, 28–30;
  chemotherapy for, 29;
  stoma, 29–30, 33, 37, 43
counseling, 19, 39, 90

depression, 4, 27, 35–38, 44, 76, 139, 174–76

deprofessionalizing, 32
diet, 6, 110, 114–15, 181–82

end of treatment, 31
endometrial cancer, 70
exercise, 6, 41, 77–80, 108, 117, 163, 181–82

fatigue, 5, 74–76, 178–79
Family and Medical Leave Act, 56
fertility preservation, 140

infertility, 138, 141, 198;
  clinics, 137, 142–45;
  chemotherapy and, 136, 139
Institute of Medicine (IOM), 128
intrusive thoughts, 12–13, 18

Kabat-Zinn, Jon, 23, 191–93

lifestyle changes, 112–13, 118
leukemia, 83, 119
lubricants, 95–97, 195–97
lymphoma, 131

menopause, 63, 86–87, 91–93, 152

National Coalition for Cancer Survivorship (NCCS), 4

Office of Cancer Survivorship, 3–4
organic food, 114

President's Cancer Panel, 3
posttraumatic stress disorder (PTSD), 41
prostate cancer, 48–49, 55

reconstructive surgery, 13–16
recurrence, 4, 17, 19, 171–73
refocusing, 20–21
relaxation, 21, 78;
    deep breathing, 21, 190;
    meditation, 22, 191–92;
    mindfulness, 22–24, 173, 191–92;
    progressive muscle, 21, 189–90

sensate focus, 100, 193–95
sexuality, 5, 129–30, 147, 179–81;
    desire for, 85
sleep, 77, 151–52, 156, 166
support groups, 14, 22
survivorship, 3
    definitions of, 3–4
Survivorship Care Plans, 6, 121–24,
    128–29, 182–83, 197

U.S. Preventive Services Task Force,
    47

work, 5, 45, 49, 52, 176–78

About the Author

Anne Katz is a clinical nurse specialist at CancerCare Manitoba. She is the author of the award-winning books *Breaking the Silence on Cancer and Sexuality: A Handbook for Health Care Providers, Woman Cancer Sex,* and *Man Cancer Sex.* She has also written *Sex When You're Sick: Reclaiming Sexual Health after Illness or Injury* and *Girl in the Know: Your Inside-and-Out Guide to Growing Up.*